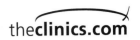

CLINICS IN PERINATOLOGY

Surfactant and Mechanical Ventilation

GUEST EDITORS
Steven M. Donn, MD
Thomas E. Wiswell, MD

D1351438

March 2007 • Volume 34 • Number 1

SAUNDERS

An Imprint of Elsevier, Inc.
PHILADELPHIA   LONDON   TORONTO   MONTREAL   SYDNEY   TOKYO

W.B. SAUNDERS COMPANY
A Division of Elsevier Inc.

Elsevier, Inc., 1600 John F. Kennedy Blvd., Suite 1800, Philadelphia, PA 19103-2899

http://www.theclinics.com

CLINICS IN PERINATOLOGY
March 2007
Editor: Carla Holloway

Volume 34, Number 1
ISSN 0095-5108
ISBN-10: 1-4160-4291-1
ISBN-13: 978-1-4160-4291-4

Clinics in Perinatology (ISSN 0095-5108) is published in quarterly by Elsevier Inc., 360 Park Avenue South, New York, NY 10010-1710. Months of issue are March, June, September, and December. Business and Editorial offices: 1600 John F. Kennedy Blvd., Suite 1800, Philadelphia, PA 19103-2899. Customer Service Office: 6277 Sea Harbor Drive, Orlando, FL 32887-4800. Periodicals postage paid at New York, NY and additional mailing offices. Subscription prices are $182.00 per year for (US individuals), $270.00 per year for (US institutions), $215.00 per year (Canadian individuals), $335.00 per year (Canadian institutions), $248.00 per year (foreign individuals), $335.00 per year (foreign institutions) $88.00 per year (US students), and $121.00 per year (foreign students). Foreign air speed delivery is included in all Clinics subscription prices. All prices are subject to change without notice. **POSTMASTER:** Send address changes to *Clinics in Perinatology*; Elsevier Periodicals Customer Service, 6277 Sea Harbor Drive, Orlando, FL 32887-4800. **Customer Service: 1-800-654-2452 (US). From outside of the US, call 1-407-345-1000.** E-mail: elspcs@elsevier.com

Clinics in Perinatology is also pubilshed in Spanish by McGraw-Hill Interamericana Editores S.A., P.O. Box 5-237, 06500 Mexico D.F., Mexico.

Clinics in Perinatology is covered in *Index Medicus, Current Contents, Excepta Medica, BIOSIS* and *ISI/BIOMED.*

Printed in the United States of America.

GUEST EDITORS

STEVEN M. DONN, MD, Professor of Pediatrics, Division of Neonatal–Perinatal Medicine, Department of Pediatrics, C.S. Mott Children's Hospital, University of Michigan Health System, Ann Arbor, Michigan

THOMAS E. WISWELL, MD, Professor of Pediatrics, Center for Neonatal Care, Florida Hospital Orlando, Orlando, Florida

CONTRIBUTORS

KABIR M. ABUBAKAR, MD, Associate Professor of Pediatrics, Division of Neonatal–Perinatal Medicine, Georgetown University, Washington DC

JUDY L. ASCHNER, MD, Professor of Pediatrics and Investigator, Department of Pediatrics and The Vanderbilt Kennedy Center, Vanderbilt University Medical Center; and Director, Division of Neonatology, Vanderbilt Children's Hospital, Nashville, Tennessee

KEITH J. BARRINGTON, MD, Director, Division of Neonatology, Neonatal Intensive Care Unit, McGill University, Royal Victoria Hospital, Montreal, Quebec, Canada

MICHAEL A. BECKER, RRT, Clinical Specialist, Department of Critical Care Services, Pediatric Respiratory Therapy, C.S. Mott Children's Hospital, University of Michigan Health System, Ann Arbor, Michigan

SHERRY E. COURTNEY, MD, MS, Division of Neonatology, North Shore Long Island Jewish Health System, New Hyde Park, New York

STEVEN M. DONN, MD, Professor of Pediatrics, Division of Neonatal–Perinatal Medicine, Department of Pediatrics, C.S. Mott Children's Hospital, University of Michigan Health System, Ann Arbor, Michigan

ANNE GREENOUGH, MD, Head of School; Professor of Neonatology and Clinical Respiratory Physiology, King's College London, Children Nationwide Regional Neonatal Intensive Care Centre, King's College Hospital, London

MARTIN KESZLER, MD, Professor of Pediatrics, Division of Neonatal–Perinatal Medicine, Georgetown University, Washington DC; and Director of Nurseries, Georgetown University Hospital, Washington DC

THIERRY LACAZE-MASMONTEIL, MD, PhD, Department of Pediatrics, Stollery Children's Hospital, University of Alberta, Edmonton, Alberta, Canada

ANDREA L. LAMPLAND, MD, Stephen J. Boros Fellow in Neonatal–Perinatal Medicine, Division of Neonatology, Department of Pediatrics, University of Minnesota, Minneapolis, Minnesota

MARK C. MAMMEL, MD, Professor of Pediatrics, Division of Neonatology, Department of Pediatrics, University of Minnesota, Minneapolis; and Director, Infant Diagnostic & Research Center, Children's Hospital of Minnesota–St. Paul, St. Paul, Minnesota

ANDRÉS MATURANA, MD, MSc, Director of Neonatology, Servicio de Neonatologia, Clinica Alemana, Vitacura; and Professor of Clinical Epidemiology, School of Medicine, Universidad del Desarrollo, Santiago, Chile

FERNANDO MOYA, MD, Director, Department of Neonatology, New Hanover Regional Medical Center and Coastal Area Health Education Center, Wilmington, North Carolina; Professor of Pediatrics, University of North Carolina, Chapel Hill, North Carolina; and Paid Consultant, Discovery Laboratories

KIRSTEN OHLER, PharmD, Department of Pharmacy Practice, University of Illinois at Chicago, Chicago, Illinois

SUBRATA SARKAR, MD, Department of Pediatrics, Division of Neonatal–Perinatal Medicine, C.S. Mott Children's Hospital, University of Michigan Health System, Ann Arbor, Michigan

ANDREAS SCHULZE, MD, Associate Professor of Pediatrics, Division of Neonatology, Dr. von Hauner Children's Hospital; Department of Obstetrics and Gynecology, Klinikum Grosshadern, Ludwig Maximilian University, Munich, Germany

JAIDEEP SINGH, MD, MRCPCH, Specialist Registrar in Neonatal Medicine, James Cook University Hospital, Middlesbrough, United Kingdom

SUNIL K. SINHA, MD, PhD, FRCP, FRCPCH, Professor of Pediatrics and Neonatal Medicine, University of Durham and James Cook University Hospital, Middlesbrough, United Kingdom

ALAN R. SPITZER, MD, Senior Vice President and Director, The Center for Research and Education, Pediatrix Medical Group, Sunrise, Florida

WIN TIN, MD, The James Cook University Hospital, Middlesbrough, UK

MICHELE C. WALSH, MD, Professor of Pediatrics, Case Western Reserve University; Director, NICU, Rainbow Babies and Childrens Hospital, Division of Neonatology, Cleveland, Ohio

THOMAS E. WISWELL, MD, Professor of Pediatrics, Center for Neonatal Care, Florida Hospital Orlando, Orlando, Florida

CONTENTS

the results has demonstrated that for the prematurely born infant who has RDS, prophylactic high-frequency oscillatory ventilation only results in a modest reduction in bronchopulmonary dysplasia, and patient-triggered ventilation (assist/control or synchronized intermittent mandatory ventilation) reduces the duration of ventilation if started in the recovery phase. Whether the newer triggered modes are more efficacious remains to be appropriately tested. In term infants who have severe respiratory failure, extracorporeal membrane oxygenation increases survival, but inhaled nitric oxide only reduces the need for extracorporeal membrane oxygenation. Research is required to identify the optimum respiratory strategy for infants who have other respiratory disorders, particularly bronchopulmonary dysplasia.

There are various causes for frequent desaturations in infants. Frequent hypoxemia is a significant change in clinical status and must be investigated carefully for possible etiology. When common extra-airway causes for desaturation are ruled out, one should attempt to distinguish between central apnea and obstructive events. The most commonly overlooked obstructive event is tracheobronchomalacia, and steps should be initiated to understand the scope of the problem through pulmonary function testing and bronchoscopy. Adequate respiratory support for the infant should be provided until adequate time passes to enable airway growth and improved cartilaginous deposition to occur. Parents must be carefully supported during this time; the stress of having an infant who requires prolonged hospitalization and care for tracheobronchomalacia is substantial.

Continuous positive airway pressure (CPAP) and noninvasive ventilation (NIV) hold much promise as means to protect the lungs of newborn infants who have respiratory distress from many causes. A wide variety of options are available to the clinician, including CPAP, bilevel CPAP, and both synchronized and unsynchronized noninvasive mechanical breaths. Limited data are available regarding the best ways to use CPAP and NIV in today's NICU environment. This article reviews current information on these modalities, including available options, possible risks, and unanswered questions.

Volume-Targeted Ventilation of Newborns

Jaideep Singh, Sunil K. Sinha, and Steven M. Donn

> Traditional management of neonatal respiratory failure has been accomplished with mechanical ventilation delivered by time-cycled, pressure-limited techniques. Although easy to use, this modality results in the delivery of tidal volumes that vary according to pulmonary compliance. In contrast, volume-targeted ventilation delivers a selected tidal volume at variable peak inspiratory pressure, resulting in consistent tidal volume delivery, even in the face of changing compliance. This article reviews salient features of volume-targeted ventilation and a review of the evidence base.

Volume Guarantee Ventilation

Martin Keszler and Kabir M. Abubakar

> Recognition that volume, not pressure, is the key factor in ventilator-induced lung injury and the association of hypocarbia with neonatal brain injury demonstrate the importance of better control delivered tidal volume. New microprocessor-based ventilator modalities combine advantages of pressure-limited ventilation with the ability to deliver a more consistent tidal volume. This article discusses automatic weaning of peak inspiratory pressure in response to changing lung compliance and respiratory effort. More consistent tidal volume, fewer excessively large breaths, lower peak pressure, less hypocapnia, shorter duration of mechanical ventilation, and lower levels of inflammatory cytokines have been documented in short-term clinical trials. It remains to be seen if these short-term benefits ultimately lead to a reduced incidence of chronic lung disease.

In Support of Pressure Support

Subrata Sarkar and Steven M. Donn

> Present generation mechanical ventilators are available with advanced microprocessor-based technology. Greater emphasis is being placed on the patient controlling the ventilator, rather than the physician controlling it. Pressure support ventilation (PSV) is a form of patient-triggered ventilation that supports spontaneous breathing during mechanical ventilation. It is flow-cycled, allowing the patient to determine the inspiratory time and rate. Each spontaneous breath is terminated when inspiratory flow decelerates to a predefined percentage of peak flow. At present, strict comparisons of the usefulness of PSV with other modalities of synchronized ventilation in newborns remain limited. This article reviews the principles and clinical applications of PSV for newborns who have respiratory failure.

The Role of High-Frequency Ventilation in Neonates: Evidence-Based Recommendations

Andrea L. Lampland and Mark C. Mammel

High-frequency ventilation (HFV) uses small tidal volumes and extremely rapid ventilator rates. Despite the wealth of laboratory and clinical research on HFV, there are no established guidelines for prioritizing the use of HFV versus conventional mechanical ventilation (CMV) in neonatal respiratory failure. Examination of the currently available randomized controlled trials and meta-analysis of HFV versus CMV does not demonstrate any clear benefit of HFV either as a primary mode or as a "rescue" mode of ventilation in neonates who have respiratory insufficiency. The current literature does support the preferential use of HFV over CMV in conjunction with inhaled nitric oxide to maximize oxygenation in hypoxemic respiratory failure, in particular, as a result of persistent pulmonary hypertension.

Animal-Derived Surfactants Versus Past and Current Synthetic Surfactants: Current Status

Fernando Moya and Andrés Maturana

In this review, the authors assess major outcomes resulting from head-to-head comparison trials of animal-derived surfactants with previous and newer synthetic surfactants and among them. They also pay special attention to issues of study design and quality of the trials reviewed. Animal-derived surfactants that contain surfactant proteins (Survanta, Infasurf, and Curosurf) perform clinically better than Exosurf, a synthetic surfactant containing only phospholipids, primarily in outcomes related to acute management of respiratory distress syndrome (RDS; faster weaning and pneumothorax) but not in overall mortality or incidence of bronchopulmonary dysplasia (BPD). Trials comparing various animal-derived surfactants that provide different amounts of surface protein B (SP-B) or phospholipids have shown minor differences in outcomes related to the management of RDS or none at all. The exception is the suggestion of better survival using a high initial dose of Curosurf when compared with Survanta. This observation is based on analysis of trials of relatively lesser quality that have included a smaller number of infants than other surfactant comparisons, however. Data from recent trials comparing a new-generation synthetic surfactant that contains a peptide mimicking the action of SP-B, Surfaxin, have shown that it performs better than Exosurf (faster weaning and less BPD) and at least as well as the animal-derived surfactants Survanta and Curosurf. The ideal surfactant comparison trial to demonstrate which surfactant is better has yet to be conducted. Future surfactant comparison trials should pay particular attention to study design, be appropriately sized, and include long-term follow-up.

GOAL STATEMENT

The goal of *Clinics in Perinatology* is to keep practicing neonatologists and maternal-fetal medicine specialists up to date with current clinical practice in perinatology by providing timely articles reviewing the state of the art in patient care.

ACCREDITATION

The *Clinics in Perinatology* is planned and implemented in accordance with the Essential Areas and Policies of the Accreditation Council for Continuing Medical Education (ACCME) through the joint sponsorship of the University of Virginia School of Medicine and Elsevier. The University of Virginia School of Medicine is accredited by the ACCME to provide continuing medical education for physicians.

The University of Virginia School of Medicine designates this educational activity for a maximum of 60 *AMA PRA Category 1 Credits*™. Physicians should only claim credit commensurate with the extent of their participation in the activity.

The American Medical Association has determined that physicians not licensed in the US who participate in this CME activity are eligible for *AMA PRA Category 1 Credits*™.

Credit can be earned by reading the text material, taking the CME examination online at http://www.theclinics.com/home/cme, and completing the evaluation. After taking the test, you will be required to review any and all incorrect answers. Following completion of the test and evaluation, your credit will be awarded and you may print your certificate.

FACULTY DISCLOSURE/CONFLICT OF INTEREST

The University of Virginia School of Medicine, as an ACCME accredited provider, endorses and strives to comply with the Accreditation Council for Continuing Medical Education (ACCME) Standards of Commercial Support, Commonwealth of Virginia statutes, University of Virginia policies and procedures, and associated federal and private regulations and guidelines on the need for disclosure and monitoring of proprietary and financial interests that may affect the scientific integrity and balance of content delivered in continuing medical education activities under our auspices.

The University of Virginia School of Medicine requires that all CME activities accredited through this institution be developed independently and be scientifically rigorous, balanced and objective in the presentation/discussion of its content, theories and practices.

All authors/editors participating in an accredited CME activity are expected to disclose to the readers relevant financial relationships with commercial entities occurring within the past 12 months (such as grants or research support, employee, consultant, stock holder, member of speakers bureau, etc.). The University of Virginia School of Medicine will employ appropriate mechanisms to resolve potential conflicts of interest to maintain the standards of fair and balanced education to the reader. Questions about specific strategies can be directed to the Office of Continuing Medical Education, University of Virginia School of Medicine, Charlottesville, Virginia.

The authors/editors listed below have identified no professional or financial affiliations for themselves or their spouse/partner:
Kabir M. Abubakar, MD; Keith J. Barrington, MD; Michael A. Becker, RRT; Carla Holloway (Acquisitions Editor); Thierry Lacaze-Masmon, MD, PhD; Andrea L. Lampland, MD; Andrés Maturana, MD, MSc; Kirsten Ohler, PharmD; Subrata Sarkar, MD; Andreas Schulze, MD; Jaideep Singh, MD, MRCPCH; Suni K. Sinha, MD, PhD, FRCP, FRCPCH; Win Tin, MD; Michele C. Walsh, MD; and, Thomas E. Winswell, MD (Guest Editor).

The authors/editors listed below identified the following professional or financial affiliations for themselves or their spouse/partner:
Judy L. Ashner, MD is on the Advisory Committee/Board for Discovery Laboratories, and has stock/ownership in Gilead Sciences.
Sherry E. Courtney, MD, MS is a consultant for Viasys, and is on the speaker's bureau and has teaching engagements for Viasys, Inc., and INO Therapeutics.
Steven M. Donn, MD (Guest Editor) is a consultant, on the speaker's bureau, and on the advisory board for Viasys Healthcare and Discovery Laboratories.
Anne Greenough, MD is on the speaker's bureau for SLE, and serves on the advisory committee/board for Abbott.
Martin Keszler, MD is an independent contractor and a consultant, and serves on the speaker's bureau, for Draeger Medical, Inc.
Mark C. Mammel, MD owns stock in United Surgical Partners, Sanofi-Aventis, Medtronic, and Nuvelo.
Fernando Moya, MD is a consultant for Discovery Laboratories and Insmed, Inc., and is on the Advisory Committee Board for Discovery Laboratories and Ferring Laboratories
Alan R. Spitzer, MD is employed by, and is a stock holder of, Pediatrix Medical Group.

Disclosure of Discussion of non-FDA approved uses for pharmaceutical products and/or medical devices:
The University of Virginia School of Medicine, as an ACCME provider, requires that all faculty presenters identify and disclose any "off label" uses for pharmaceutical and medical device products. The University of Virginia School of Medicine recommends that each physician fully review all the available data on new products or procedures prior to instituting them with patients.

TO ENROLL

To enroll in the Clinics in Perinatology Continuing Medical Education program, call customer service at 1-800-654-2452 or visit us online at www.theclinics.com/home/cme. The CME program is available to subscribers for an additional fee of $195.00

FORTHCOMING ISSUES

RECENT ISSUES

ELSEVIER
SAUNDERS

Clin Perinatol 34 (2007) xiii

CLINICS IN
PERINATOLOGY

Erratum

Mass Spectrometry in Neonatal Medicine and Clinical Diagnosis—The Potential Use of Mass Spectrometry in Neonatal Brain Monitoring

In the September 2006 issue of *Clinics in Perinatology*, an error appears on pages viii and 729 in the title of Drs. Alan R. Spitzer and Donald Chace's article. The correct article title is "Mass Spectrometry in Neonatal Medicine and Clinical Diagnosis—The Potential Use of Mass Spectrometry in Neonatal Brain Monitoring."

CLINICS IN
PERINATOLOGY

Clin Perinatol 34 (2007) xv–xvi

Preface

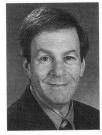 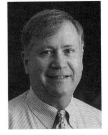

Steven M. Donn, MD   Thomas E. Wiswell, MD
Guest Editors

It has been nearly 6 years since we were first invited to edit an edition of *Clinics in Perinatology*, entitled "Update on Mechanical Ventilation and Exogenous Surfactant." We were honored when Saunders asked us to reprise the edition. Much has transpired as technology and bioengineering continue to change the therapeutic options in neonatal ICUs.

In choosing the topics and the authors for the current edition, we have tried to balance a desire to present innovative care with evidence-based medicine. The proliferation of new ideas, diagnostics, and treatments has been so rapid that infusion into mainstream care often precedes or even precludes adequate testing during the time of equipoise. Nevertheless, instituting even the most innovative of therapies without sufficient assessment of safety and efficacy in our fragile population is a disservice to patients and their families.

We have assembled an "all-star team" of clinical investigators who are the leaders in their respective areas of interest and who have made significant contributions to the field of neonatal pulmonary care. We have asked each of them to present the available evidence and to critically review the literature pertinent to their articles. Several of the topics originally were reviewed in the 2001 edition and are updated. For instance, the article dealing with pulmonary graphics has taken its illustrations from a next-generation ventilator graphic monitor, and the articles dealing with surfactant therapy include areas not addressed previously. Neonatal demographics also are a moving target, with increasing numbers of tiny survivors who have significant morbidity. The volume concludes with a provocative article focusing

doi:10.1016/j.clp.2007.01.002   *perinatology.theclinics.com*

on the need to define optimum long-term outcome measures if the quality of survival is to improve.

We would like to thank all of the authors for their efforts in producing this edition. All have worked diligently to provide a balanced picture and to examine the need for further investigation in many areas. We appreciate the vote of confidence from Saunders in asking us to edit a second edition, and we hope the readership also will find it worthwhile.

Steven M. Donn, MD
Division of Neonatal-Perinatal Medicine
Department of Pediatrics
C.S. Mott Children's Hospital
University of Michigan Health System
1500 E. Medical Center Drive
Ann Arbor, MI 48109, USA

E-mail address: smdonnmd@med.umich.edu

Thomas E. Wiswell, MD
Center for Neonatal Care
Florida Hospital Orlando
2718 North Orange Avenue, Suite B
Orlando, FL 32804, USA

E-mail address: Thomas_Wiswell@yahoo.com

CLINICS IN
PERINATOLOGY

Clin Perinatol 34 (2007) 1–17

Real-Time Pulmonary Graphic Monitoring

Michael A. Becker, RRT[a], Steven M. Donn, MD[b],*

[a]Department of Critical Care Services, Pediatric Respiratory Therapy,
C.S. Mott Children's Hospital, University of Michigan Health System, 1500 E. Medical
Center Drive, Ann Arbor, MI 48109-0254, USA
[b]Division of Neonatal–Perinatal Medicine, Department of Pediatrics,
F5790 C.S. Mott Children's Hospital/0254, University of Michigan Health System,
1500 E. Medical Center Drive, Ann Arbor, MI 48109-0254, USA

Until recently, the use of neonatal bedside real-time graphic monitoring was either nonexistent or tedious at best. For a quarter of a century, the mainstay of neonatal mechanical ventilation was continuous flow, time-cycled, pressure-limited ventilation without patient synchronization of the ventilator breaths. Primary parameter adjustments with this modality included the mandatory respiratory rate, peak inspiratory pressure (PIP), positive end expiratory pressure (PEEP), inspiratory time, and circuit flow rate. The assessment of the appropriateness of these parameters was determined subjectively by noting color, observing chest excursions, and listening to breath sounds, and objectively by intermittent assessment of gas exchange and radiography. The advent of transcutaneous PO_2 and PCO_2 monitoring, as well as pulse oximetry, provided evidence that the management of neonatal respiratory failure is a dynamic process requiring much more intensive surveillance than the intermittent assessments.

In the late 1980s, pulmonary mechanics technology was finally made available in the neonatal intensive care unit (NICU). This portable equipment was brought to the bedside and used by specially trained individuals. The objective was to be able to assess diseases, evaluate medication treatments such as bronchodilators, and to adjust the ventilator parameters to achieve optimal ventilation and oxygenation. The principle device used to obtain the bedside pulmonary mechanics was a pneumotachograph. However, it needed to be disassembled, cleaned, and reassembled between

---

* Corresponding author.
E-mail address: smdonnmd@med.umich.edu (S.M. Donn).

0095-5108/07/$ - see front matter © 2007 Elsevier Inc. All rights reserved.
doi:10.1016/j.clp.2006.12.002

patients. This process was long and tedious and if not done correctly could affect the accuracy of the measurements. Testing also required disconnecting and reconnecting the patient from the ventilator, which often disturbed the baby and changed the pattern of breathing. The pneumotachograph was heavy and bulky and if not supported appropriately could change the position of the endotracheal tube in small infants. It added significant deadspace to the ventilator circuit and increased the work of breathing. The values obtained were basic; they were generally tidal volume, compliance, and resistance. Although probably reasonably accurate, the values supplied the practitioner with limited information, which was merely a "snapshot" of the patient's pulmonary status and interaction with the ventilator. The information was generally not useful in determining events that occurred either before or after the study.

Today, real-time bedside pulmonary graphics have become a standard of care in most—if not all—NICUs. Most of the new generation of mechanical ventilators incorporate proximal airway sensors, also referred to as transducers, that are positioned between the ventilator circuit and the endotracheal tube. They are extremely light and introduce minimal additional deadspace. This microprocessor-based technology is integral to the intended function of the ventilator. The more common sensor technologies fall into one of two categories: thermal or differential pressure type. The sensor detects either flow or pressure and converts the signal to a clinically useful analog value. For example, the flow signal can be integrated to obtain a volume measurement. The sensor also is used to detect patient effort to facilitate or "trigger" synchrony between the patient's own effort and the delivery of a mechanical breath by the ventilator. The information is presented in real-time and is a continuous display, not the snapshot of the previous pulmonary function technology but more similar to a "motion picture" of each individual breath as well as trends of measured values over an extended period of time.

Graphic monitoring assists the clinician at the bedside in several ways. It can be helpful in fine-tuning or adjusting ventilator parameters. For instance, one can track and determine the progress of a disease such as respiratory distress syndrome by following compliance measurements. Graphic monitoring may help to determine the patient's response to pharmacologic agents such as surfactant, diuretics, or bronchodilators. The clinician also has the ability to trend monitored events over a prolonged period of time.

The understanding of graphic monitoring may at times be considered complex. There are many clinical situations that may be identified at the bedside. Each patient is different and provides unique learning experiences. This being said, if the clinician becomes comfortable with identifying a small number of common situations, it may greatly enhance clinical expertise.

All of the examples provided were obtained using the AVEA ventilator (VIASYS Healthcare, Yorba Linda, California). Graphic displays were downloaded using a commercially available software package (VGA2USB, Epiphan Systems, Inc., Ottawa, Ontario, Canada). The AVEA monitor uses a four-color display, making it easy to distinguish between inspiration and expiration, and spontaneous and mechanical breaths. To create black and white figures, a negative of the color image was made and then converted to black and white using gray-scale technology.

Although space limitations preclude the authors publishing an extensive atlas of neonatal pulmonary graphics, there are several comprehensive texts and reviews to which the reader is referred [1–4]. The authors will instead stress principles and some of the more important clinical applications.

Pulmonary wave forms

The three major wave forms are pressure, volume, and flow. These wave forms are displayed versus time. It is important that the vertical axis be properly scaled so that the uppermost and lowermost portions of the wave forms are included on the display. Fig. 1 shows a typical representation of these wave forms.

Pressure wave form

The pressure wave form has upward (inspiration) and downward (expiration) scalars. If PEEP is used, the wave form will begin and end at

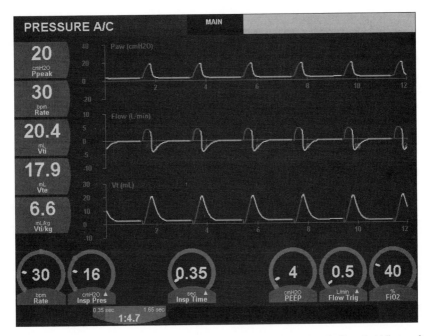

Fig. 1. Pulmonary wave forms. These include the pressure (*upper panel*), flow (*middle panel*), and volume (*lower panel*) wave forms displayed versus time.

this value and not reach zero. The uppermost point of the wave form represents PIP, whereas the area under the curve is the mean airway pressure. The inspiratory time can be measured from the point of upward deflection until PIP is reached; expiratory time begins at PIP and lasts until the next positive deflection. The total cycle time is the interval from the origin of one upward deflection until the start of the next.

Oxygenation is a function of mean airway pressure. Thus, increasing the area under the curve will improve oxygenation. This can be accomplished by increases in PIP, PEEP, inspiratory time, and to a lesser extent, the rate (Figs. 2–5). Ventilation is a function of tidal volume and frequency. The primary determinant of tidal volume is amplitude, the difference between PIP and PEEP, often referred to as ΔP. Thus, to enhance ventilation, consider changes in amplitude (higher PIP, lower PEEP, or both) and increases in ventilator frequency and/or expiratory time (Figs. 6 and 7).

Flow wave form

The flow wave form is the most difficult to understand and interpret, probably because it has two separate components. Anything *above* the zero baseline represents positive flow, or in other words, gas flow *into* the patient, and thus *inspiration*. Inspiratory flow has two components: accelerating flow (at the start of inspiration), and decelerating flow (velocity slows as the lung approaches capacity). The highest point of the positive point of the wave form is *peak inspiratory flow*. Anything *below* the zero baseline represents negative flow, or gas flow *from* the patient, and thus *expiration*. The expiratory flow wave form similarly has two components: accelerating flow (at the start of expiration), and decelerating flow (velocity slows as the lung empties to functional residual capacity). The lowest negative point of the wave form is *peak expiratory flow*.

Fig. 8 demonstrates a potentially dangerous situation. This is gas trapping, whereby incomplete emptying of the lung occurs. Note that before the decelerating expiratory wave form reaches the baseline (a zero flow state), the accelerating inspiratory flow wave of the subsequent breath begins. Thus, more gas is entering the lung than is leaving it. Ultimately, this can create overdistension, inadvertent PEEP, and alveolar rupture leading to pneumothorax or pulmonary interstitial emphysema. Clinical

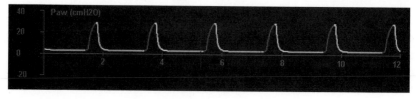

Fig. 2. Note the change in the area under the pressure wave form compared with Fig. 1, brought about by increasing the peak inspiratory pressure.

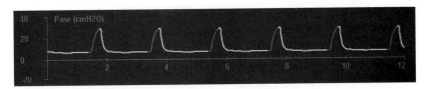

Fig. 3. Note the change in the area under the pressure wave form compared with Fig. 2, brought about by increasing the positive end expiratory pressure.

considerations aimed at alleviating this condition could be: (1) decreasing the set respiratory rate; (2) decreasing the inspiratory time to give more expiratory time; and (3) if the patient is triggering the respiratory rate, consider that the tidal volume is not appropriate (too small) and the patient may be experiencing hypoventilation, or the patient may be hypoxemic and attempt to increase mean airway pressure by creating a higher PEEP. In this case, an increase in the PEEP level may be appropriate.

The flow wave form may help distinguish breath types. Pressure-targeted ventilation produces a spiked or sinusoidal wave form (Fig. 9), whereas volume-targeted ventilation produces a characteristic square wave whereby flow plateaus and is held constant (Fig. 10). Some newer ventilators can also produce a decelerating volume wave form (Fig. 11).

Volume wave form

The volume wave form is similar in appearance to the pressure wave form, except that it should start and end on the baseline. The shape of the pressure wave form demonstrates how volume is delivered to the baby. During pressure-targeted ventilation, peak volume delivery occurs early in inspiration, then decreases. This is in contrast to volume-targeted ventilation, which creates a "shark's fin" pressure wave form, whereby peak volume delivery occurs at the end of inspiration.

Pulmonary mechanics and loops

Pulmonary mechanics can also be assessed when changes in pressure versus volume or flow versus volume are graphed over time. Fig. 12 demonstrates a typical display of pressure–volume and flow–volume loops.

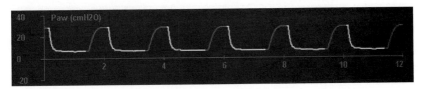

Fig. 4. Note the change in the area under the pressure wave form compared with Fig. 3, brought about by increasing the inspiratory time.

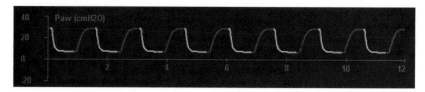

Fig. 5. Note the change in the area under the pressure wave form compared with Fig. 4, brought about by increasing the ventilator rate.

Pressure–volume loop

The pressure–volume loop begins at PEEP. As the pressure delivered to the lung increases, there is a concomitant increase in the volume of gas delivered to the lung. The inspiratory limb ends at PIP, and the expiratory or deflationary limb begins, whereby pressure and volume fall as the lung empties. The shape of this loop is referred to as *hysteresis* and describes the mechanical properties of the lung as it is filled and emptied. If an imaginary line is drawn to connect the origin of the loop with the PIP, it can estimate the dynamic compliance of the lung. Compliance is mathematically determined by the change in volume divided by the change in pressure and is graphically displayed on the LOOP screen. Visually (if data are appropriately scaled), a loop indicating good compliance will be described as upright (compliance axis > 45°), and a loop indicating poor compliance is described as flat, or lying on its side.

Distortions in the pressure–volume loop may indicate disturbances in lung mechanics. A common issue before tidal volume measurement was available was lung overinflation, which occurs when the ventilator delivers volume that exceeds lung capacity, resulting in excess pressure without an increase in volume. A loop that flattens at the upper end, often referred to as either a "duck tail" or "penguin beak" (Fig. 13), indicates hyperinflation, whereby the incremental delivery of pressure results in little or no further volume delivery. Inadequate hysteresis, producing a narrow loop, may be indicative of inadequate flow (Fig. 14).

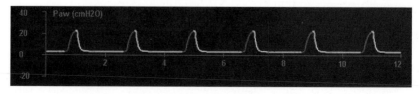

Fig. 6. Note the change in the amplitude of the pressure wave form, compared with Fig. 1, brought about by increasing the peak inspiratory pressure.

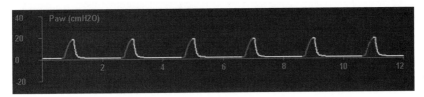

Fig. 7. Note the change in the amplitude of the pressure wave form, compared with Fig. 1, brought about by decreasing the positive end expiratory pressure.

Flow–volume loop

The flow–volume loop describes changes in these parameters over the inspiratory (positive) and expiratory (negative) phases of the respiratory cycle. A normal flow–volume loop should be circular or oval in appearance. The upper and lower limits, representing peak inspiratory and expiratory flows, respectively, should be nearly equivalent. One caveat needs to be stressed: although pressure–volume loops can only be drawn one way, flow–volume loops may be drawn in several ways. Unfortunately, there is as yet no agreement among the device manufacturers, so it becomes incumbent upon the users to determine how each device draws the loop. This is most easily accomplished by first determining which half is inspiration and which half is expiration, then connecting the two.

The flow–volume loop allows us to make inferences regarding resistance. If resistance is high, there will be an impedance to flow, resulting in a smaller volume of gas flow over a constant time.

Figs. 15 and 16 show the effect of altering resistance by use of a bronchodilator. The reference loop (see Fig. 15) has a normal configuration, but both the peak inspiratory and peak expiratory flows are low. After treatment, resistance improves, and there is a demonstrable difference in the appearance of the loop (see Fig. 16).

The flow–volume loop can help to differentiate increases in inspiratory and expiratory resistance. This may be of both diagnostic (eg, suspecting a vascular ring) and therapeutic (eg, need for high PEEP) benefit. Increased resistance to flow is seen in several disease processes. Examples may be meconium aspiration syndrome or bronchopulmonary dysplasia. This may

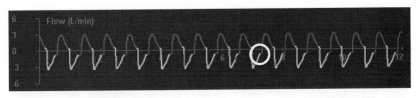

Fig. 8. Flow wave form demonstrates gas trapping. The decelerating expiratory limb fails to reach the baseline before the next breath begins (circled), preventing complete emptying of the lung.

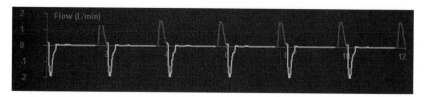

Fig. 9. The sinusoidal pressure wave form is characteristic of pressure-targeted ventilation.

be observed on both the LOOP and WAVE screens. On the LOOP screen there is a low flow rate. On the WAVE screen there is a prolonged decelerating expiratory phase and a slower return to baseline (Fig. 17).

Other clinical considerations

Endotracheal tube leaks

Another common finding seen on both the flow–volume and pressure–volume loops is the presence of an endotracheal tube leak. This is common in neonates because cuffed endotracheal tubes are not used. The amount of leak is the difference in the measured inspiratory and expiratory tidal volumes. Leaks prevent the normal "closure" of the pressure–volume loop; the expiratory limb just "hangs." On the flow–volume loop, the expiratory portion of the loop reaches the volume axis before the origin (Fig. 18). Leaks may also be suspected by looking at the volume wave form, whereby the expiratory portion also fails to reach the baseline.

Patient triggering and synchronization is now an important feature of neonatal ventilation. Most ventilators have an adjustable triggering threshold so that the clinician can compensate for a leak in the system. If the sensitivity is not set correctly, autocycling may occur (the ventilator misinterprets the leak, which creates a flow signal, as spontaneous effort by the patient and delivers a mechanical breath). Fig. 19 is an example of the WAVE screen during autocycling. Note the rhythmic breaths without a pause and the large leak (volumes not returning to baseline) on the volume wave form.

Optimum positive end expiratory pressure

Graphics can aid in the determination of the best PEEP. Fig. 20 shows an abnormality in the pressure–volume loop, characterized by a need for

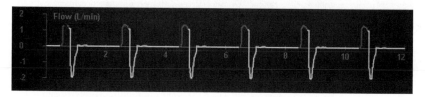

Fig. 10. Volume-targeted ventilation produces a square wave, with a flow plateau.

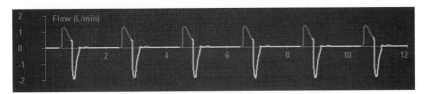

Fig. 11. Some newer ventilators provide the option of selecting a decelerating volume wave form.

a higher opening pressure. The loop looks "box-like" rather than elliptical. Note the improvement when the PEEP (and concomitantly the PIP) is raised (Fig. 21). Alternatively, choosing the PEEP and PIP that produce the best compliance is another way to achieve this.

Turbulence

Turbulence can be created if the circuit airway flow is set too high, or if there are secretions in the airway, sensor, or circuit that interfere with laminar flow and create a noisy signal. This can be seen on both wave forms (Fig. 22) and loops (Fig. 23). It generally indicates a need for careful inspection for secretions or condensation, consideration for endotracheal tube suctioning, as well as an evaluation of the appropriateness of the flow rate.

Pressure support

Pressure support ventilation is generally used in conjunction with synchronized intermittent mandatory ventilation. It supports spontaneous breaths. Graphics are helpful in distinguishing the two populations of breaths and allows for independent adjustments based on the patient's response and inherent respiratory rate (Fig. 24).

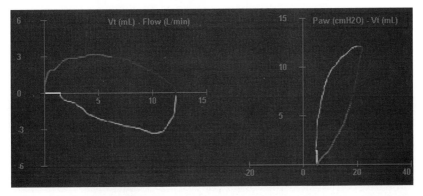

Fig. 12. Typical display of pulmonary loops. On the left is the pressure–volume loop, with pressure on the abscissa and volume on the ordinate. On the right is the flow–volume loop, with volume on the abscissa and flow on the ordinate.

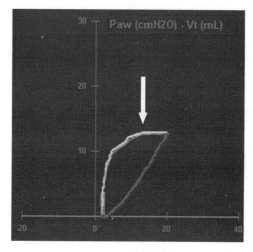

Fig. 13. Pressure–volume loop demonstrating hyperinflation. Note the flat portion of the volume curve (*arrow*), where much less volume is recruited over the last few increments in pressure.

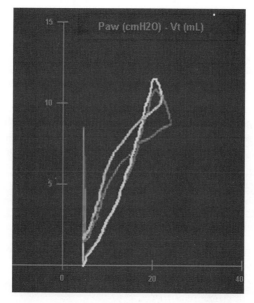

Fig. 14. Pressure–volume loop demonstrating inadequate hysteresis. There is little separation between the inflationary and deflationary limbs. Air hunger creates the "figure-eight" appearance at the end of inspiration.

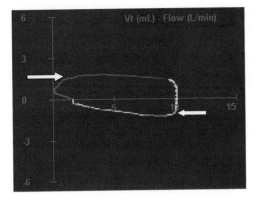

Fig. 15. Flow-volume loop in a patient who had elevated resistance. Note peak inspiratory and expiratory flows (*arrows*).

Flow-cycling

Cycling is the mechanism by which inspiration is initiated and terminated. Traditional pressure-limited ventilation was time-cycled, whereby inspiration ended after a preset time, chosen by the clinician. Transducer and microprocessor-based technology now gives the clinician the option of flow-cycling, whereby inspiration ends not according to time, but according to an airway flow change. During inspiration, the ventilator records the peak inspiratory flow rate and subsequently terminates inspiration when decelerating inspiratory flow decays to a small percentage of peak flow, usually 5% to 10%. This enables not only inspiratory synchrony, whereby the baby triggers the breath, but expiratory synchrony, because the mechanical breath is terminated just before the patient is about

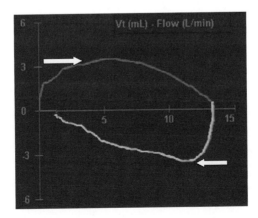

Fig. 16. Flow–volume loop in a patient who had a good therapeutic response to bronchodilator therapy. Note the improvement in peak flows (*arrows*), compared with those in Fig. 16.

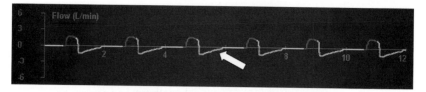

Fig. 17. Increased expiratory resistance diminishes the slope of the decelerating expiratory flow
wave form, increasing the time to reach the baseline (*arrow*).

to end his or her own respiratory effort. Flow-cycling is important during
assist/control ventilation. It prevents inversion of the inspiratory/expiratory
ratio, which occurs when the inspiratory time is fixed and expiratory time is
sacrificed. Figs. 25 and 26 demonstrate the difference between time-cycling
and flow-cycling. Note how the flow wave form transitions directly into
expiration and does not pause at the baseline zero flow state during
flow-cycling.

Trend data

There can be considerable clinical value in the assessment of events over
time. Relevant respiratory parameters can be presented in two forms:
numerically or as a chart (Fig. 27). This can be extremely helpful in
determining alterations in ventilator support, changes in disease processes,
and response to treatments such as surfactant. All information is stored
over a 24-hour period for review by the clinician. It can also be downloaded
for preservation.

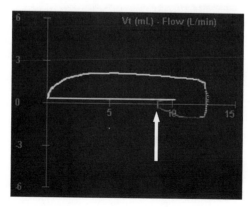

Fig. 18. Large endotracheal tube leak. Note that the expiratory portion of the flow-volume
loop fails to reach the origin (*arrow*).

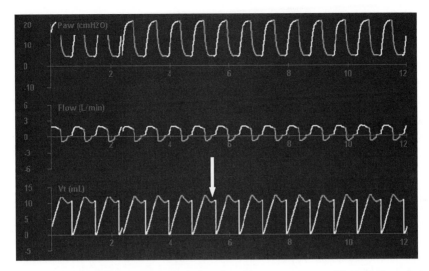

Fig. 19. Autocycling. Note the rhythmic breaths without a pause as well as the large leak (volume wave form does not return to the baseline; *arrow*).

Summary

Although there is truly no substitute for clinical assessment at the bedside of a mechanically ventilated infant, real-time pulmonary graphics do provide useful information regarding the breath-to-breath performance of

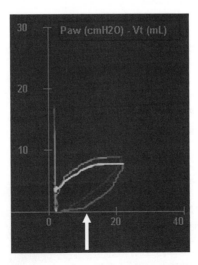

Fig. 20. Determining the optimum PEEP. This pressure–volume loop demonstrates poor compliance (note the "side-lying" appearance) and the need for a higher opening pressure. No volume recruitment occurs until a considerable portion of the inflationary limb has occurred (*arrow*).

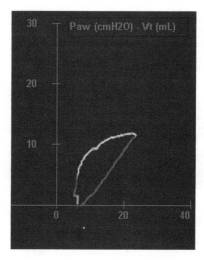

Fig. 21. Determining the optimum PEEP. Increasing the PEEP (and concomitantly the PIP) normalize the configuration of the pressure–volume loop and improve the compliance.

the ventilator and its interaction with the baby. Some complications of mechanical ventilation, such as gas trapping and hyperinflation, may be detected by graphics before they are clinically apparent. Fine-tuning of ventilator settings based on pathophysiology and patient response can replace "ventilation by rote" and allow for customization of settings. Continuous monitoring can also decrease the frequency of blood gas analysis and

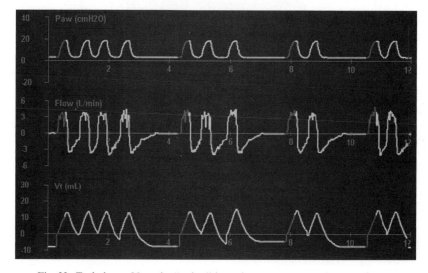

Fig. 22. Turbulence. Note the "noisy," irregular appearance to the wave forms.

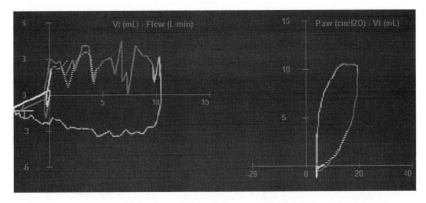

Fig. 23. Turbulence. Note the "noisy," irregular appearance to the loops.

radiography, reducing the cost of care and increasing the comfort of the patient.

Users must have a satisfactory knowledge of how the devices work, how to troubleshoot them, and when to be circumspect about the information provided. There is no true evidence base as yet to determine cost-effectiveness or clinical efficacy, but the time is right to begin such investigations. Can a baby be managed with a sophisticated, multimodal mechanical ventilator without pulmonary graphics? Probably, but it would be a lot like using a computer without its monitor.

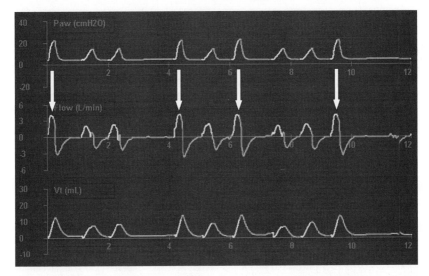

Fig. 24. Pressure support ventilation. Wave forms help to distinguish mandatory breaths (providing full support; *arrows*), from pressure-supported spontaneous breaths, set to deliver partial support.

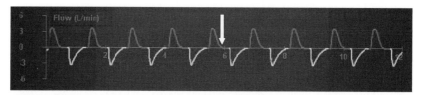

Fig. 25. Time-cycled ventilation. Note how the decelerating portion of the inspiratory flow wave form comes down all the way to the baseline (*arrow*).

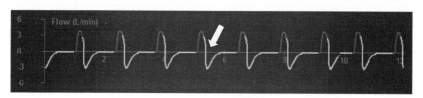

Fig. 26. Flow-cycled ventilation. Note how the decelerating inspiratory flow wave form transitions directly into expiration (*arrow*). This is because inspiratory flow is terminated at a certain percentage of peak flow, rather than by time.

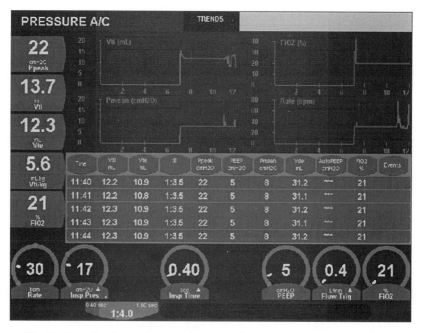

Fig. 27. Example of a trend screen, showing various selected parameters over time.

References

[1] Bhutani VK, Sivieri EM. Pulmonary function and graphics. In: Goldsmith JP, Karotkin EH, editors. Assisted ventilation of the neonate. 4th edition. Philadelphia: Saunders/Elsevier; 2003. p. 293–309.

[2] Donn SM, editor. Neonatal and pediatric pulmonary graphics: principles and clinical applications. Armonk (NY): Futura Publishing Co; 1998.

[3] Nicks JJ. Neonatal graphic monitoring. In: Donn SM, Sinha SK, editors. Manual of neonatal respiratory care. 2nd edition. Philadelphia: Mosby/Elsevier; 2006. p. 134–47.

[4] Sinha SK, Nicks JJ, Donn SM. Graphic analysis of pulmonary mechanics in neonates receiving assisted ventilation. Arch Dis Child 1996;75:F213–8.

ELSEVIER
SAUNDERS

CLINICS IN
PERINATOLOGY

Clin Perinatol 34 (2007) 19–33

Respiratory Gas Conditioning and Humidification

Andreas Schulze, MD[a,b,*]

[a]Division of Neonatology, Dr. von Hauner Children's Hospital, Munich, Germany
[b]Department of Obstetrics and Gynecology, Klinikum Grosshadern, Ludwig Maximilian
University, Marchioninistr. 15, D-81377, Munich, Germany

Although there have been great advances in our understanding of pulmonary pathophysiology in the management of neonatal lung disorders, the proper humidification and conditioning of delivered gas remains a mystery to most clinicians managing these devices. This article attempts to unravel the mystery and describe the physiologic bases for humidification and gas conditioning.

Basic physics of heat and humidity

Medical grade gases have virtually no water content at room temperature. There are three options to deliver water into inspired gas or directly into the airways:

Vaporization of water using heated humidifiers or heat and moisture exchangers ("artificial noses").
Nebulization of water using jet or ultrasonic devices.
Periodic instillation of bolus water or normal saline solution into the endotracheal or tracheostomy tube as is commonly done prior to suctioning procedures.

Fundamental differences exist between nebulized and vaporized water. Nebulization creates a dispersion of small droplets of water in air. These particles may vary in size from about 0.5 to 5 μm. They are visible as mist because they scatter light and may carry infectious agents or other particulate matter.

* Division of Neonatology and Department of Obstetrics and Gynecology, Klinikum Grosshadern, Ludwig Maximilian University, Marchioninistr. 15, D-81377 Munich, Germany.
    E-mail address: andreas.schulze@med.uni-muenchen.de

In contrast, vaporization generates a molecular (ie, gaseous) distribution of water in air. Water vapor is thus invisible and unable to carry infectious agents. It exerts a gaseous pressure, which amounts to a partial pressure of water of 47 mm Hg when air is fully saturated with water vapor at 37°C. This corresponds to a water vapor mass of 44 mg of water per liter of gas. The partial pressure of water vapor at saturation depends solely on the temperature. The fraction of water vapor pressure at saturation, 37°C, and 760 mm Hg ambient pressure is therefore $F_{H_2O} = 47$ mm Hg/760 mm Hg $= 0.062$ (6.2%). The term absolute humidity (AH) is defined as the amount of water vapor (in milligrams) per gas volume (in liters) at a given temperature. Relative humidity (RH) is the actual water vapor content of the gas volume (in milligrams) relative to the water vapor content (in milligrams) of this same gas volume at saturation at the same temperature. There is a fixed relationship between AH, RH, and temperature (Fig. 1).

Air takes up energy when nebulized water or liquid water is converted into water vapor. Conversely, heat is generated in the process of rainout of water vapor (condensation). There are two components to the total energy content of air: a sensible and a latent heat content. The air temperature solely reflects the former, whereas the water vapor mass reflects the latter. It is important to understand that changing the air temperature alone without changes in water vapor mass constitutes a small change in total energy content compared with changing the humidity of the gas. The difference may approach an order of magnitude. Warming of frigid inspiratory air does little cooling to the upper airway lining compared with the amount of heat loss that occurs when this air is particularly dry. Conversely, if air is inhaled at 39°C without being fully saturated with water vapor, it quickly cools to core body temperature without significant heating of the airway lining. The

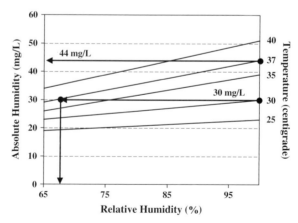

Fig. 1. The relative humidity of a gas depends on its absolute water content and gas temperature. At 37°C and 100% relative humidity, the respiratory gas has 44 mg/L absolute water content. If the gas is saturated (100% relative humidity) at 30°C, its water content is only 30 mg/L. When the gas is then warmed to 37°C, its relative humidity falls to less than 70%.

following example illustrates this issue quantitatively. If air is saturated with water vapor at 37°C in a humidifier chamber and subsequently dry heated to 39°C in a heated breathing circuit, this dry heating adds almost no energy to the gas. It contains 143 J/g at 37°C, 100% relative humidity versus 145 J/g at 39°C, 90% relative humidity. If, however, air enters the airway at much higher than core body temperature and full saturation, there may be a risk for thermal injury.

Structure and function of the airway lining

The lining of the respiratory tract consists of three layers: a basal cellular layer, an aqueous (sol) layer, and a viscoelastic gel (mucus) layer at the luminal surface. Most of the upper airways and the entire tracheobronchial tree down to the respiratory bronchioles are covered by ciliated epithelial cells. Each cell carries about 200 cilia at its apex. The cilia are 5 to 6 μm in length and carry a crown of short claws at their tip. When extended, the cilia may reach through the aqueous layer and get their claws entangled with the macromolecular network of the mucus, which floats at the surface of the aqueous layer. A movement cycle of a single cilium consists of two parts. During the effective stroke, the fully extended cilium moves in a plane approximately perpendicular to the cell surface and pulls the mucus layer forward. It then bends down toward the cell surface, thereby disengaging from the gel layer, and swings back near the surface of the cell to reach its starting position (recovery stroke through a less viscous medium). Under normal circumstances, the orientation of the effective strokes is always such that the mucus is propelled in a cephalad direction. Neighboring cilia beat in a coordinated fashion so that waves of aligned cilia move through the airway lining fluid. There are various other specific cell types, such as serous cells and Clara cells, in the cellular layer of the airway lining, each of which may be concerned with a specific function [1]. Mucus is secreted by goblet cells and submucosal mucous glands as globules of 1 to 2 μm in diameter. They absorb water from the aqueous layer and subsequently swell rapidly. Mucus consists of glycoproteins, proteoglycans, lipids, and 95% water [2]. It forms small flakes [3], larger plaques, or blanket-like covers [4,5] that float on the luminal surface and trap inhaled particles and other compounds, such as bacteria, macrophages, and cell debris [6]. Experimental evidence exists that mucus secretion is stimulated when particles come into contact with the ciliated surface. Such particles are subsequently encapsulated by mucus and carried away by the ciliary escalator [7]. The structure and function of the various components of this intricate system may easily become disturbed when the inspired gas is inadequately conditioned in infants who have an artificial airway.

Inspired gas conditioning in the respiratory tract

The alveolar air is fully saturated with water vapor at core body temperature, whereas ambient air is cooler and contains less water. This gradient in heat and water vapor pressure is maintained under physiologic conditions along the nose and upper airways [8]. They function as a counter-current heat and moisture exchanger. The inspired air gains heat and water vapor from the upper airway lining, which is partly recovered when the expired gas loses heat and water condenses back to the airway surface. This recovery occurs because the upper airway temperature remains below core body temperature during expiration. Breathing is associated with a net heat and water loss because the expired air temperature is higher than ambient temperature under normal circumstances [9]. The greater this difference in temperature between the inspired and expired gas, the higher are the losses. They must be replenished by the airway epithelium, which in turn is supplied by the bronchial circulation. It is entirely unclear under which circumstances the capacity of the airway lining to humidify cold and dry gas becomes overcharged. This capacity is likely different in healthy and diseased states. Water transport through the mucosa itself into the aqueous layer of the airway lining is possibly rate limiting. Another potential limitation of water supply to the airway lining may result from decreased blood perfusion to the mucosa. It was suggested that this occurs when cold air is inhaled and mucosal blood vessels constrict in a response similar to the reduction in skin perfusion in a cold environment [10]. It could be argued teleologically that keeping the upper airway cool during expiration by restricting blood flow facilitates heat and water recovery. It has been shown in hyperventilated anesthetized dogs, however, that tracheobronchial blood flow increases with breathing cold or warm dry air [11]. This response is not mediated by the autonomic nervous system [12].

The level at which the inspired air reaches core body temperature and full saturation with water vapor is called the isothermic saturation boundary [13]. It is located at the level of the main stem bronchi in the adult during normal quiet breathing of room air [14]. Its position varies with the heat and moisture content of the inspired air and depends on the pattern of breathing. For example, it moves cephalad with slow and shallow breathing [15], and oral breathing moves it downward compared with nasal breathing [16]. Incompletely conditioned air may penetrate deep into the distal parts of the tracheobronchial tree during high minute ventilation of frigid air because of the large volume of air to be conditioned and the short residence time at any given point [14,17]. Bypassing the upper airway (for example, by using a tracheostomy tube) also is associated with a much greater burden for humidification on the distal airways. Overall, however, under normal physiologic circumstances only a small segment of the airway surface is exposed to a temperature below core body temperature and less than full saturation with water vapor.

Risks of using poorly conditioned medical gases in infants who have an artificial airway

The optimal temperature and humidity of the inspired gas for infants undergoing mechanical ventilation has been a matter of controversy. Also, the minimal acceptable level of temperature and humidity has not been clearly established by clinical studies. International and United States standards recommend an absolute humidity level of inspired gas greater than 33 mg/L in patients whose supraglottic airway is bypassed [18–20]. There is no doubt that inadequate humidification may lead to progressive airway dysfunction and systemic effects, depending on the degree of under-humidification and coolness, the exposure time, and the underlying disease.

The mucociliary transport system is probably the most sensitive respiratory function to changes in inspired gas humidity and temperature [21]. Transport velocity depends on mucus rheology, the depth of the aqueous airway lining layer, and cilia beat frequency. Dry inspired gas changes the viscosity gradient of the airway lining. Dehydrated mucus slows the transport rate and cilia beat frequency. Thinning of the aqueous layer impairs the recovery stroke of cilia [22,23]. The mucociliary machinery may recover with rehumidification after short periods of desiccation. Cessation of cilia activity for 3 hours is irreversible, however, and is followed by inflammation and sloughing of the mucosa [24]. Such damage deprives the upper airway of its function as a heat and moisture exchanger. Subsequently, the isothermic saturation boundary retreats into smaller airways and the area of damaged mucosa progressively extends into the periphery of the lung.

Because the depth of the airway lining fluid is only about 7 to 12 μm [25], water loss by evaporation may increase the osmolarity. This increase may induce bronchial smooth muscle contraction in patients who have exercise-induced asthma independently of the inhaled air temperature [26–29]. The mechanism by which a change in the osmotic environment can lead to bronchoconstriction is unknown. Airway irritant receptors have been implemented as possible mediators. It is also unknown whether a critical threshold of respiratory water loss exists to induce a stimulus for bronchoconstriction, or whether this mechanism occurs in preterm infants who have chronic lung disease.

In a retrospective study, mechanically ventilated infants weighing less than 1500 g at birth had significantly more air leaks and more severe chronic lung disease if exposed during their first 4 days of life to inspired gas less than 36.6°C and with less than 37 mg H_2O/L [30]. This association could not be corroborated for more mature infants, suggesting that the resistance to poor inspiratory gas conditioning might be a function of gestational age. The cause of necrotizing tracheobronchitis in mechanically ventilated infants and adults has not been fully elucidated, but it is rational to assume that inadequate humidification is a significant contributor [31–33].

The mucociliary elevator moves secretions up to the tip of the endotracheal tube. This material accumulates and resides there for a variable period of time awaiting removal by suctioning. It is subjected to desiccation by any inspiratory gas leaving the endotracheal tube with a capacity to accommodate more water vapor. Inspissation is faster the lower the humidity and the higher the airflow at the endotracheal tube outlet. High minute ventilation and an endotracheal tube leak hasten this process. It has been suggested that humidity levels below a critical threshold of 31 mg H_2O/L are associated with a high risk for endotracheal tube plugging in infants [34]. At least theoretically, however, this does not imply that any humidity level above this threshold and below full saturation at core body temperature is safe in regard to upper airway obstruction by inspissated secretions.

Mechanical ventilation with dry gas results in a mean decrease in rectal temperature by 1.4°C within one hour in neonates. Even moderate warming to 31.5°C and humidifying the inspiratory gas reduces the insensible water loss in intubated preterm infants significantly and consistently to levels below those of extubated infants in room air at 27°C [35].

Severe underhumidification finally leads to impaired surfactant activity, decreased functional residual capacity, atelectasis, and compromised pulmonary mechanics [36].

Devices for inspiratory gas conditioning and humidification procedures

Heated humidifiers

For various physiologic reasons, it is rational to deliver the inspiratory gas to endotracheally intubated infants at or close to core body temperature and full saturation. Heated humidifiers (Fig. 2) can achieve this goal. The respiratory gas is warmed inside the humidification chamber to a set target temperature and water vapor is added from the heated water reservoir. Inspiratory circuit tubing containing a heated wire is then used to maintain or slightly raise the gas temperature to prevent water rainout before the gas reaches the infant. At a set humidifier chamber temperature of 37°C, the gas absorbs 44 mg/L of water, which corresponds to full saturation (100% RH) unless the vaporizing capacity is low relative to the size of the gas flow. The vaporizing capacity of the humidification chamber depends on its water surface area and temperature. Recording the water consumption of the chamber over time is a simple test to check for sufficient vaporization. Because most infant ventilators use continuous circuit flow of known rate, the absolute and relative humidity delivered at the chamber outlet can be calculated from the humidifier's water consumption rate. Any decrease in gas temperature along the way from the humidification chamber to the wye adaptor induces condensation if the gas was saturated at the chamber outlet. This implies that if the chamber temperature was set at or below 37°C, any rainout in the tubing indicates moisture loss from the respiratory gas. The gas reaching the infant is underhumidified. It must be emphasized that rainout in the inspiratory limb of the ventilator circuit does not indicate proper humidification in such situations. To the contrary, condensation is necessarily associated with underhumidification. The inspiratory gas can rapidly cool in unheated segments of the circuit. This cooling is promoted by the large outer surface area of small diameter tubing

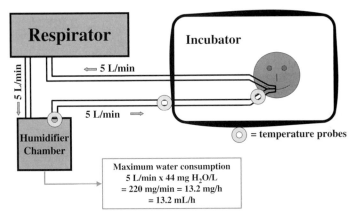

Fig. 2. Position of three temperature probes of a heated-wire humidification system for infants. The user sets the target temperature to be reached at the endotracheal tube adaptor. This temperature is commonly set at or slightly greater than 37°C. The temperature inside the humidifier chamber must be high enough to vaporize an amount of water near the absolute water content of gas saturated at 37°C (44 mg/L). The water consumption rate of a humidifier chamber required to reach a target respiratory gas humidity can be calculated from the circuit flow rate. Observation of this water consumption rate can be used as a simple test of the efficiency of a humidifier.

(particularly when corrugated), by drafts around the tubing (air conditioned rooms), and by low room temperatures. The decrease in temperature is larger with smaller circuit gas flow rates because of the longer contact time. Insulating unheated segments of the inspiratory circuit may partly obviate these problems. Rainout should also be avoided for other reasons. Condensate is easily contaminated, may be flushed down the endotracheal tube (with risks of airway obstruction and nosocomial pneumonia), and may disturb the function of the ventilator. In a regular application for an intubated subject, therefore, a heated humidifier should be set up with a chamber temperature of 37°C to saturate the gas with 44 mg/L of water. To avoid loss of moisture in the inspiratory limb of the heated circuit, the target gas temperature at the wye adaptor can be set at 39°C so that the gas arrives with slightly less than full saturation. The gas quickly cools to core body temperature inside the adapter and the endotracheal tube.

The technology required for preterm infants is slightly more complex because the ventilator circuit passes through two different environments: the room and the incubator or radiant warmer. The temperature probe close to the patient connection serves to monitor the respiratory gas temperature. It is commonly part of a servo-control, which aims to maintain the set gas temperature at the wye adaptor by controlling the circuit's heated wire power output. If the temperature probe is in the presence of a heated field, it may register a temperature higher than the actual respiratory gas temperature as a result of radiation or convection from the warmer environment. This may signal to the servo to decrease the heating output of the ventilator circuit and lead to loss of gas temperature and rainout. Such a problem may arise when the incubator temperature is higher than the targeted gas temperature or from a radiation heat source. Insulating the temperature probe by a light reflective patch or other material can improve the performance of the system. Another way to alleviate this problem is to place the temperature probe just outside the heated field and use an unheated extension adaptor tubing to carry the gas through the heated field to the infant. The extension tube does not need to incorporate heated wires because its temperature is maintained by the heated field. If cooler incubator temperatures are used (as usually used for older preterm infants), rainout occurs in the unheated segment, particularly at low circuit gas flow rates. A circuit should then be used that is equipped with a heated wire along the entire length of its inspiratory limb. Another suitable type of circuit is that with two temperature probes, one outside the heated field and the other close to the wye adaptor. These circuits can perform well over a range of incubator temperatures both greater than and less than the target respiratory gas temperature. This is because the heated wire servo-control can be programmed to select the lower of the two recorded temperatures to drive the power output. The maximum heat output of any heated wire circuit may not be sufficient to meet target gas temperatures under extremes of room and incubator temperatures. Also, generic circuits have been on the market that may not be fully compatible with the humidifier and its power source. There has been a warning that covering heated wire circuits with drapes or other material for insulation may involve a risk for melting or charring of circuit components [37].

Artificial noses

Heat and moisture exchangers (HMEs) are designed to recover part of the heat and moisture contained in the expired air. A sponge material of low thermal conductivity inside the clear plastic housing of these devices absorbs heat and condenses water vapor during expiration for subsequent release during inspiration. HMEs are an attractive alternative to heated humidifiers for several reasons, such as simplification of the ventilator circuit, passive operation without requirement of external energy and water sources, no ventilator circuit condensate, low risk for circuit contamination [38], and low expense. Additionally, some HMEs are coated with bacteriostatic substances and equipped with bacterial or viral filters (HMEF). Devices called hygroscopic condenser humidifiers (HCHs) use hygroscopic compounds, such as $CaCl_2$, $MgCl_2$, LiCl, or others, to increase the water retention capacity. Small HME/HCHs for neonatal applications are commercially available, but data on their use are sparse. Theoretically, an application in small subjects may be particularly effective because mean delivered inspiratory humidity increases inversely with tidal volume [39]. Also, the HME membranes may become saturated before a large volume expiration has been completed, which increases respiratory water loss. A pediatric HME maintained an average inspiratory humidity greater than 30 mg/L in a clinical study involving neonates for a test period of 6 hours [40]. Other clinical studies on pediatric and neonatal application confirmed the ability of HME/ HCHs to conserve heat and to provide humidity levels that are appropriate for short-term conventional mechanical ventilation [41–43]. Bench studies on high-frequency oscillatory ventilation in a neonatal lung model showed that a neonatal HME was able to provide more than 35 mg/L of mean humidity at the proximal end of the endotracheal tube adapter. The HME dampened the oscillatory pressure amplitude less than a neonatal endotracheal tube of 3.5 mm inner diameter [44]. The safety and effectiveness of HME/HCH for long-term mechanical ventilation is controversial in adults [45–49] and has not been established in infants. Depending on their actual water load and duration of use, HMEs add a variable resistance and dead space to the circuit [50–52]. A risk for airway occlusion from clogging with secretions or from a dislodgement of HME internal components [53] has been reported for infants even during short-term application. Also, an expiratory air leak impairs the barrier effect against moisture loss [54,55]. HME must not be used in conjunction with heated humidifiers, nebulizers, or metered dose inhalers, which may cause a hazardous increase in device resistance [56] or wash off the hygroscopic coating [57]. Different brands of HME/HCHs may vary widely in their performance characteristics. Their effectiveness is not reliably reflected by indirect clinical measures, such as the occurrence of nosocomial pneumonia, number of endotracheal tube occlusions, or frequency of tracheal suctioning and instillation [58]. Visual evaluation of the amount of moisture in the adapter segment between the endotracheal tube and the HME/HCH was found to closely correlate with objective measurements of the delivered humidity, however [59]. Device performance has improved much during recent years, and further advances can be expected to facilitate neonatal applications. Microprocessor-controlled active release of additional external heat and water into the airway between an HME and the endotracheal tube adapter increased the inspired gas humidity to 100% at 37°C without obvious untoward effects in 24-hour studies in adults. Such hybrid systems, however, require further study and refinement [60].

Aerosol application

Aerosol water particles that range in size from about 1 to 10 μm may deposit on the airway by impaction (larger particles) or sedimentation (smaller particles). Sedimentation occurs as a gravitational effect when airflow velocity declines in the smaller airways. An aerosol cannot contribute to respiratory gas conditioning downstream to the isothermic saturation boundary because the gas is already fully saturated. For this same reason, aerosol water particles cannot be eliminated in this airway region through evaporation and exhalation. They therefore become a water burden on the mucosa that needs to be absorbed by the airway epithelium to maintain an appropriate periciliary fluid depth. An increase in depth of the airway lining's aqueous layer may make it impossible for the cilia to reach the mucous layer and thus impair mucus transport. Furthermore, if the aerosol deposition rate exceeds absorption capacity, this may lead to increased airway resistance [61,62] and possibly narrowing or occlusion of small airways. Severe systemic overhydration subsequent to ultrasonic aerosol therapy has been described in a term newborn infant [63], and similar occurrences have been reported in adults [64]. If an aerosol stream meets the airway proximal to the isothermic saturation boundary, the particulate water can theoretically contribute to the gas conditioning process by evaporation before and after deposition. The droplets, however, contain only sensible heat and the mucosa needs to supply most of the latent heat for vaporization. This process cools the airway. If the inspiratory gas is supplied through the endotracheal tube at body core temperature and close to full saturation, the isothermic saturation boundary is located near the tip of the endotracheal tube. In such a situation, any aerosol may contribute little, if anything, to appropriate gas conditioning. Water or normal saline nebulization, therefore, seems to offer no significant benefit for inspiratory gas conditioning and may entail a risk for overhumidification [65].

Irrigation of the airway

It is common clinical practice to instill small amounts of water or normal saline solution into the endotracheal tube before suctioning procedures in the belief that this provides moisture and loosens tenacious secretions. A randomized controlled trial showed a lower endotracheal tube resistance and fewer hemorrhagic secretions when periodic bolus instillation of normal saline solution was used before suctioning in adults on mechanical ventilation with HMEs [66]. It has been shown, however, that more than 80% of the instillate may remain inside the airway after suctioning and probably later is absorbed or removed by the mucociliary system [67]. Suggested amounts of fluid to be used in infants vary widely from 0.1 mL/kg to 0.5 mL [37]. The safety and effectiveness of this practice, under conditions of appropriate warming and humidification of respiratory gases, remain dubious [68].

Inspiratory gas conditioning and the nosocomial infection risk

Water vapor as such cannot transmit an infection. It has been shown, however, that cold water and hot water humidifier chambers, reservoirs of nebulizers, ventilator circuits, and circuit condensate may all become colonized with infectious agents [69–71]. Theoretically, the airway may then become contaminated from colonized condensate flushed inadvertently into the airway, from colonized aerosol particles, and directly from a colonized circuit. A bubble-through humidifier chamber may not only produce water vapor but also some aerosol capable of dispersing infectious particles. The colonization risk may be reduced by the use of sterile closed delivery systems or by maintaining a water reservoir temperature greater than 60°C (pasteurization) [36]. It has been shown in adults, however, that such colonization usually originates from the patient's own respiratory flora and may occur within a few hours of connecting a sterile circuit [72,73]. It was subsequently observed that the incidence of nosocomial pneumonia in adults was not increased when ventilator circuits were changed less frequently than every 24 hours or even between patients [50,74,75]. Nevertheless, although these studies indicate that ventilator circuit changes may be extended to more than 48 hours, the optimal rate of circuit changes for infants is unknown. Changing a ventilator circuit is not a benign procedure because it may disrupt ventilation in a potentially dangerous way, and medical personnel may become a vector for cross-contamination between patients [76]. Arguments can therefore be made for weekly circuit changes or for no circuit changes at all, except between patients.

In 2005, a meta-analysis of randomized controlled trials found a protective effect against ventilator-associated pneumonia in adults with the use of HMEs compared with heated humidifiers, particularly in patients ventilated for 7 days or longer [77]. The size of this effect, however, is likely small; it could not be corroborated in two more recent studies on a large number of patients [50,78].

Summary

There is a strong physiologic rationale for delivering the inspiratory gas at or close to core body temperature and saturated with water vapor to infants who have an artificial airway undergoing longer-term mechanical ventilatory assistance. Cascade humidifiers with a heated wire ventilatory circuit may achieve this goal safely. Whenever saturated air leaves the humidifier chamber at 37°C and condensate accumulates in the circuit, the gas loses humidity and acquires the potential to dry airway secretions near the tip of the endotracheal tube. Heat and moisture exchangers and hygroscopic condenser humidifiers with or without bacterial filters have become available for neonates. They can provide sufficient moisture output for short-term ventilation without excessive additional dead space or flow-resistive loads for term infants. Their safety and efficacy for very low birthweight infants and for long-term mechanical ventilation have not been established conclusively. A broader application of these inexpensive and simple devices is likely to occur with further design improvements. When heated humidifiers are appropriately applied, water or normal saline aerosol application offers no additional significant advantage in inspiratory gas conditioning and may impose a water overload on the airway or even systemically. Although airway irrigation by periodic bolus instillation of normal saline solution before suctioning procedures is widely practiced in neonatology, virtually no data exist on its safety and efficacy when used with appropriately humidified inspired gas. There is no evidence that conditioning of inspired gas to core body temperature and full water vapor saturation may promote nosocomial respiratory infections.

References

[1] Jeffery PK, Reid LM. The respiratory mucus membrane. In: Brain JD, Proctor DF, Reid LM, editors. Respiratory defense mechanisms. Part I. New York: Marcel Dekker; 1977. p. 193–245.

[2] Yeager H. Tracheobronchial secretions. Am J Med 1971;50:493–501.

[3] Iravani J, van As A. Mucus transport in the tracheobronchial tree of normal and bronchitic rats. J Pathol 1972;106:81–93.

[4] Aiello E, Sleigh MA. Ciliary function of the frog oropharyngeal epithelium. Cell Tissue Res 1977;178:267–8.

[5] Puchelle E, Petit A, Adnet JJ. Fine structure of the frog palate mucociliary epithelium. J Submicrosc Cytol 1984;16:273–82.

[6] Brain JD, Godlaski JJ, Sorokin SP. Quantification, origin and fate of pulmonary macrophages. In: Brain JD, Proctor DF, Reid LM, editors. Respiratory defense mechanisms. Part II. New York: Marcel Dekker; 1977. p. 849–92.

[7] Spungin B, Silberberg A. Stimulation of mucus secretion, ciliary activity and transport in frog palate epithelium. Am J Physiol 1984;247:C299–308.

[8] Rouadi P, Baroody FM, Abbott D, et al. A technique to measure the ability of the human nose to warm and humidify air. J Appl Physiol 1999;87:400–6.

[9] Walker JEC, Wells RE, Merrill EW. Heat and water exchange in the respiratory tract. Am J Med 1961;30:259–67.

[10] McFadden ER. Respiratory heat and water exchange: physiological and clinical implications. J Appl Physiol 1983;54:331–6.

[11] Baile EM, Dahlby RW, Wiggs DR, et al. Role of tracheal and bronchial circulation in respiratory heat exchange. J Appl Physiol 1985;58:217–22.

[12] Baile EM, Osborne S, Pare PD. Effect of autonomic blockade on tracheobronchial blood flow. J Appl Physiol 1987;62:520–5.

[13] Dery R, Pelletier J, Jacques A, et al. Humidity in anaesthesiology. 3. Heat and moisture patterns in the respiratory tract during anaesthesia with the semi-closed system. Can Anaesth Soc J 1967;14:287–98.

[14] McFadden ER, Pichurko BM, Bowman HF, et al. Thermal mapping of the airways in humans. J Appl Physiol 1985;58:564–70.

[15] Dery R. The evolution of heat and moisture in the respiratory tract during anaesthesia with a non-rebreathing system. Can Anaesth Soc J 1973;20:296–309.

[16] Primiano FP, Saidel GM, Montague FW, et al. Water vapor and temperature dynamics in the upper airways of normal and CF subjects. Eur Respir J 1988;1:407–14.

[17] McFadden ER, Dension DM, Waller JR, et al. Direct recordings of the temperatures in the tracheobronchial tree in normal man. J Clin Invest 1982;69:700–5.

[18] American Society for Testing and Materials. Standard specification for humidifiers for medical use. ASTM F1690-96 (2004).

[19] Miyoshi E, Fujino Y, Uchiyama A, et al. Effects of gas leak on triggering function, humidification, and inspiratory oxygen fraction during noninvasive positive airway pressure ventilation. Chest 2005;128:3691–8.

[20] International Organization for Standardization. Humidifiers for medical use. ISO 8185 (1997).

[21] Williams R, Rankin N, Smith T, et al. Relationship between the humidity and temperature of inspired gas and the function of the airway mucosa. Crit Care Med 1996;24:1920–9.

[22] Puchelle E, Zahm JM, Quemada D. Rheologic properties controlling mucociliary frequency and respiratory mucus transport. Biorheology 1987;24:557–63.

[23] Sleigh MA, Blake JR, Liron N. The propulsion of mucus by cilia. Am Rev Respir Dis 1988; 137:726–41.

[24] Hirsch JA, Tokayer JL, Robinson MJ, et al. Effects of dry air and subsequent humidification on tracheal mucus velocity in dogs. J Appl Physiol 1975;39:242–6.

[25] Kilburn KH. A hypothesis for pulmonary clearance and its implications. Am Rev Respir Dis 1968;98:449–63.

[26] Anderson SD, Schoeffel RE, Black JL, et al. Airway cooling as the stimulus to exercise-induced asthma—a re-evaluation. Eur J Respir Dis 1985;67:20–30.

[27] Anderson SD, Schoeffel RE, Follet R, et al. Sensitivity to heat and water loss at rest and during exercise in asthmatic patients. Eur J Respir Dis 1982;63:459–71.

[28] Freed AN, Anderson SD, Daviskas E. Thermally induced asthma and airway drying. Am J Respir Crit Care Med 2000;161:2112–3.

[29] Hahn A, Anderson SD, Morton AR, et al. A reinterpretation of the effect of temperature and water content of the inspired air in exercise-induced asthma. Am Rev Respir Dis 1984;130: 575–9.

[30] Tarnow-Mordi WO, Reid E, Griffiths P, et al. Low inspired gas temperature and respiratory complications in very low birth weight infants. J Pediatr 1989;114:438–42.

[31] Boros SJ, Mammel MC, Lewallen PK, et al. Necrotizing tracheobronchitis: a complication of high frequency ventilation. J Pediatr 1986;109:95–100.

[32] Circeo LE, Heard SO, Griffiths E, et al. Overwhelming necrotizing tracheobronchitis due to inadequate humidification during high-frequency jet ventilation. Chest 1991;100: 268–9.

[33] Hanson JB, Waldstein G, Hernandez JA, et al. Necrotizing tracheobronchitis. Am J Dis Child 1988;142:1094–8.

[34] Lomholt N, Cook R, Lunding M. A method of humidification in ventilator treatment of neonates. Br J Anaesth 1968;40:335–40.

[35] Sosulski R, Polin RA, Baumgart S. Respiratory water loss and heat balance in intubated infants receiving humidified air. J Pediatr 1983;103:307–10.

[36] Shelly MP, Lloyd GM, Park GR. A review of the mechanisms and methods of humidification of inspired gases. Intensive Care Med 1988;14:1–9.

[37] Quinn W, Sandifer L, Goldsmith JP. Pulmonary care. In: Goldsmith JP, Karotkin EH, editors. Assisted ventilation of the neonate. 3rd edition. Philadelphia: W.B. Saunders; 1996. p. 101–23.

[38] Dreyfuss D, Djedaini K, Gros I, et al. Mechanical ventilation with heated humidifiers or heat and moisture exchangers: effects on patient colonization and incidence of nosocomial pneumonia. Am J Respir Crit Care Med 1995;151:986–92.

[39] Mebius C. A comparative evaluation of disposable humidifiers. Acta Anaesthesiol Scand 1983;27:403–9.

[40] Schiffmann H, Rathgeber J, Singer D, et al. Airway humidification in mechanically ventilated neonates and infants: a comparative study of a heat and moisture exchanger vs. a heated humidifier using a new fast-response capacitive humidity sensor. Crit Care Med 1997;25: 1755–60.

[41] Bissonnette B, Sessler DI. Passive or active inspired gas humidification increases thermal steady-state temperatures in anesthetized infants. Anesth Analg 1989;69:783–7.

[42] Bissonnette B, Sessler DI, LaFlamme P. Intraoperative temperature monitoring sites in infants and children and the effect of inspired gas warming on esophageal temperature. Anesth Analg 1989;69:192–6.

[43] Bissonnette B, Sessler DI, LaFlamme P. Passive and active inspired gas humidification in infants and children. Anesthesiology 1989;71:350–4.

[44] Schiffmann H, Singer S, Singer D, et al. Determination of airway humidification in high-frequency oscillatory ventilation using an artificial neonatal lung model. Comparison of a heated humidifier and a heat and moisture exchanger. Intensive Care Med 1999;25:997–1002.

[45] Branson RD, Davis K Jr, Campbell RS, et al. Humidification in the intensive care unit. Prospective study of a new protocol utilizing heated humidification and a hygroscopic condenser humidifier. Chest 1993;104:1800–5.

[46] Kollef MH, Shapiro SD, Boyd V, et al. A randomized clinical trial comparing an extended-use hygroscopic condenser humidifier with heated-water humidification in mechanically ventilated patients. Chest 1998;113:759–67.

[47] Misset B, Escudier B, Rivara D, et al. Heat and moisture exchanger vs. heated humidifier during long-term mechanical ventilation. A prospective randomized study. Chest 1991; 100:160–3.

[48] Nakagawa NK, Macchione M, Petrolino HM, et al. Effects of a heat and moisture exchanger and a heated humidifier on respiratory mucus in patients undergoing mechanical ventilation. Crit Care Med 2000;28:312–7.

[49] Ricard JD, Le Miere E, Markowicz P, et al. Efficiency and safety of mechanical ventilation with a heat and moisture exchanger changed only once a week. Am J Respir Crit Care Med 2000;161:104–9.

[50] Boots RJ, George N, Faoagali JL, et al. Double-heater-wire circuits and heat-and-moisture exchangers and the risk of ventilator-associated pneumonia. Crit Care Med 2006;34:687–93.

[51] Briassoulis G, Paraschou D, Hatzis T. Hypercapnia due to a heat and moisture exchanger. Intensive Care Med 2000;26:147.

[52] Iotti GA, Olivei MC, Palo A, et al. Unfavorable mechanical effects of heat and moisture exchangers in ventilated patients. Intensive Care Med 1997;23:399–405.

[53] Casta A, Houck CS. Acute intraoperative endotracheal tube obstruction associated with a heat and moisture exchanger in an infant. Anesth Analg 1997;84:939–40.

[54] Gedeon A, Mebius C, Palmer K. Neonatal hygroscopic condenser humidifier. Crit Care Med 1987;15:51–4.

[55] Tilling SE, Hayes B. Heat and moisture exchangers in artificial ventilation. An experimental study of the effect of gas leakage. Br J Anaesth 1987;59:1181–8.

[56] Barnes SD, Normoyle DA. Failure of ventilation in an infant due to increased resistance of a disposable heat and moisture exchanger. Anesth Analg 1996;83:193.

[57] Rathgeber J, Züchner K, Burchardi H. Conditioning of air in mechanically ventilated patients. In: Vincent JL, editor. Yearbook of intensive care and emergency medicine. Berlin: Springer; 1996. p. 501–19.

[58] Djedaini K, Markowicz P, Mier L, et al. Comparisons between three types of heat and moisture exchangers changed every 48 hours during mechanical ventilation. Am J Respir Crit Care Med 1997;155:A769.

[59] Ricard JD, Markowicz P, Djedaini K, et al. Bedside evaluation of efficient airway humidification during mechanical ventilation of the critically ill. Chest 1999;115:1646–52.

[60] Larsson A, Gustafsson A, Svanborg L. A new device for 100 per cent humidification of inspired air. Crit Care 2000;4:54–60.

[61] Cheney FW, Butler J. The effects of ultrasonically produced aerosols on airway resistance in man. Anesthesiology 1968;29:1099–106.

[62] Melville GN, Josenhans WT, Ulmer WT. Changes in specific airway resistance during prolonged breathing of moist air. Can J Physiol Pharmacol 1970;48:592–7.

[63] Tamer MA, Modell JH, Rieffel CN. Hyponatremia secondary to ultrasonic aerosol therapy in the newborn infant. J Pediatr 1970;77:1051–4.

[64] Sladen A, Laver MB, Pontoppidan H. Pulmonary complications and water retention in prolonged mechanical ventilation. N Engl J Med 1968;279:448–53.

[65] Williams RB. The effects of excessive humidity. Respir Care Clin N Am 1998;4:215–28.

[66] Tenaillon A, Boiteau R, Humbert M, et al. Effect of periodical instillation of isotonic salt solute on tracheal tubes permeability. Intensive Care Med 1990;16:S112.

[67] Hanley MV, Rudd T, Butler J. What happens to intratracheal saline instillations. Am Rev Respir Dis 1978;117:124S.

[68] Ackerman MH. The use of bolus normal saline instillations in artificial airways: is it useful or necessary. Heart Lung 1985;14:505–6.

[69] Christopher KL, Saravolatz LD, Bush TL, et al. The potential role of respiratory therapy equipment in cross infection. A study using a canine model for pneumonia. Am Rev Respir Dis 1983;128:271–5.

[70] Craven DE, Goularte TA, Make BJ. Contaminated condensate in mechanical ventilator circuits: a risk factor for nosocomial pneumonia. Am Rev Respir Dis 1984;129:625–8.

[71] Redding PJ, McWalter PW. Pseudomonas fluorescence cross infection due to contaminated humidifier water. Br Med J 1980;281:275.

[72] Craven DE, Connolly MG, Lichtenberg DA, et al. Contamination of mechanical ventilators with tubing changes every 24 or 48 hours. N Engl J Med 1982;306:1505–9.

[73] Lareau SC, Ryan KJ, Diener CF. The relationship between frequency of ventilator circuit changes and infectious hazard. Am Rev Respir Dis 1978;118:493–6.

[74] Dreyfuss D, Djedaini K, Weber P, et al. Prospective study of nosocomial pneumonia and of patient and circuit colonization during mechanical ventilation with circuit changes every 48 hours versus no change. Am Rev Respir Dis 1991;143:738–43.

[75] Hess D, Burns E, Romagnoli D, et al. Weekly ventilator circuit changes. A strategy to reduce costs without affecting pneumonia rates. Anesthesiology 1995;82:903–11.

[76] Cadwallader HL, Bradley CR, Ayliffe GA. Bacterial contamination and frequency of changing ventilator circuitry. J Hosp Infect 1990;15:65–72.

[77] Kola A, Eckmanns T, Gastmeier P. Efficacy of heat and moisture exchangers in preventing ventilator-associated pneumonia: meta-analysis of randomized controlled trials. Intensive Care Med 2005;31:5–11.

[78] Lacherade JC, Auburtin M, Cerf C, et al. Impact of humidification systems on ventilator-associated pneumonia: a randomized multicenter trial. Am J Respir Crit Care Med 2005;172:1276–82.

CLINICS IN
PERINATOLOGY

Clin Perinatol 34 (2007) 35–53

Matching Ventilatory Support Strategies to Respiratory Pathophysiology

Anne Greenough, MD[a],*,
Steven M. Donn, MD[b]

[a]Division of Asthma, Allergy and Lung Biology, King's College London,
Children Nationwide Regional Neonatal Intensive Care Centre,
4th Floor, Golden Jubilee Wing, King's College Hospital,
London SE5 9PJ, UK
[b]Department of Pediatrics, Division of Neonatal–Perinatal Medicine,
C.S. Mott Children's Hospital, University of Michigan Health System,
1500 E. Medical Center Drive, Ann Arbor,
MI 48109-0254, USA

During the last two decades, new respiratory techniques have become available to support the neonate. Although these have been actively researched, many studies have only included prematurely born infants who have acute respiratory distress. The newborn can suffer from various diseases, each with a different pathophysiology and impact on lung function. A term infant who has meconium aspiration syndrome may have over-distended lungs with high airway resistance, whereas the surfactant-deficient lungs of prematurely born infants are atelectatic and noncompliant. Thus, the concept of "one size fits all" can no longer be an appropriate management strategy, and the results of studies examining the efficacy of respiratory support modes that have included only one type of lung disorder may not be generalized to others.

In this review, the authors discuss respiratory strategies according to pathophysiology and critically evaluate the evidence, because many of the studies undertaken have lacked suitable or indeed any comparator controls, and other randomized trials have been too small to robustly test a clinically meaningful outcome.

AG has received research grants and/or support to attend meetings from SLE Systems UK, Draeger Medical, and F. Stephan Biomedical.
* Corresponding author.
E-mail address: anne.greenough@kcl.ac.uk (A. Greenough).

Techniques

Time-cycled, pressure-limited ventilation

Time-cycled, pressure-limited ventilation (intermittent positive pressure ventilation [IPPV]) has been the most frequently used mode for the newborn. During IPPV, inflations can be delivered at rates of 30 to 120 bpm; when rates of 60 bpm or more are used, this is termed *high-frequency positive pressure ventilation* (HFPPV). Inspiratory times between 0.3 and 0.5 seconds with a longer expiratory than inspiratory time (giving a physiologic inspiratory/expiratory ratio) are generally used, because these are similar to spontaneous respiratory times in the preterm infant and more likely to promote a synchronous interaction and improved gas exchange [1,2]. If, however, the infant has severe disease, an inspiratory time longer than the expiratory time is sometimes used (reversed inspiratory/expiratory ratio) to increase mean airway pressure (MAP) and oxygenation. Positive end expiratory pressures (PEEP) of 3 to 6 cmH_2O are generally employed, but if the infant has severe disease, the PEEP can be raised as high as 12 cmH_2O, again to increase MAP. The relative effectiveness of these variations, except for comparing different rates (see later discussion), have usually only been tested in physiologic studies with gas exchange as the outcome.

Patient-triggered ventilation

Patient-triggered ventilation was reintroduced into neonatal intensive care in the 1980s, initially as assist/control (A/C) (inflations triggered by every spontaneous breath that exceed the critical trigger threshold) and synchronized intermittent mandatory ventilation (SIMV) (only the preset number of inflations are triggered regardless of the infant's spontaneous respiratory rate). Newer triggered modes, such as pressure support ventilation (PSV) and proportional assist ventilation (PAV), are now available. During PSV, not only the initiation (as with A/C and SIMV), but also the termination of ventilator inflation are determined by the infant's spontaneous respiratory efforts by using airway flow changes as an expiratory trigger. Inflation is terminated when the inspiratory flow level reaches a certain percentage of peak flow. For example, in PSV mode of the Draeger Babylog 8000 (Draeger Medical, Luebeck, Germany), inflation is terminated when the flow is reduced to 15% of the maximum inspiratory flow, whereas PSV termination criteria used with the VIP BIRD (Bird Products, Palm Springs, California) are 5% to 25%, depending on the delivered tidal volume. This is referred to as *flow cycling*. During PAV, the applied pressure is servo-controlled throughout each spontaneous breath, and the frequency, timing, and rate of lung inflation are controlled by the patient. The applied pressure increases in proportion to the tidal volume and inspiratory flow generated by the patient. This can be enhanced to reduce the work of breathing [3].

Volume-targeted ventilation

Many ventilator types designed for use in neonates can deliver a preset tidal volume; this ventilator modality will subsequently be referred to as *volume-targeted ventilation* (VTV). During VTV, a set tidal volume is delivered despite changes in the infant's respiratory compliance and/or efforts; this is achieved by servo-controlled adjustments in the inflating pressure. The adjustments in inflating pressure are made in response to differences in the preset and either the exhaled or inhaled volume. There are different forms of VTV [4]. During volume-controlled or volume-support ventilation, the desired tidal volume is selected and the duration of inflation depends on the time taken for the volume to be delivered, which is adjusted by changes in the inspiratory flow rate. During Volume guarantee (Draeger Medical, Luebeck, Germany) ventilation, a preset expiratory tidal volume is selected, but the preset inspiratory time determines the duration of inflation, and the maximum pressure set by the clinician limits the maximum peak inflation pressure. The desired tidal volume, however, will not be delivered if the preset peak inspiratory pressure is too low or there is no positive pressure plateau. There is also volume-limited ventilation, during which the pressure support for any inflation is aborted if the measured inspired tidal volume exceeds a preset upper limit. During volume-controlled inflation, there is breath-by-breath servo-controlled flow, which is constant during inspiration so that the required volume is delivered over the set inspiratory time. Ventilator manufactures have used different strategies to achieve VTV. The SLE 5000 (Specialised Laboratory Equipment Ltd., UK) and Bear Cub 750 psv (Viasys Healthcare, Palm Springs, California) deliver targeted tidal or volume-limited ventilation, the Draeger Babylog 8000 delivers volume guarantee ventilation, the VIP BIRD and Avea (Viasys Healthcare, Palm Springs, California) deliver volume-controlled (or volume-support) ventilation and the Stephanie paediatric ventilator (F. Stephan Biomedical, Germany) delivers volume-controlled inspiration. In clinical studies, volume guarantee (VG) levels between 4 and 6 mL/kg have been used, but there is evidence to suggest that the VG level used may be critical to efficacy. In one study [5], a VG level of 4 mL/kg with SIMV in the first 48 hours after birth was associated with avoidance of hypocarbia and hypercarbia only 90% of the time. It seems likely that 6 mL/kg may be the most appropriate level. A level of 6 but not 4.5 mL/kg reduced the duration of hypoxemic episodes during SIMV in one study [6], and in another trial, 6 mL/kg compared with 4 or 5 mL/kg was associated with the lowest work of breathing [7]. Both VTV and VG are described in more detail in other articles in this issue.

High-frequency ventilation

Forms of high-frequency ventilation include high-frequency jet ventilation (HFJV), high-frequency flow interruption (HFFI), and high-frequency oscillatory ventilation (HFOV). HFJV is a modification of the technique initially developed to provide respiratory support during bronchoscopy. A high-pressure source is used to deliver short bursts of gas through a small-bore injector cannula in a specially designed endotracheal tube, or alternatively through a special proximal endotracheal tube adapter. The pulses are superimposed on a constant flow (PEEP) provided by a tandem conventional ventilator, which may also be used to deliver periodic sigh breaths. Frequencies between 150 and 660/min are used with short (eg, 20 msec) inspiratory times. During HFFI, small volumes of gas at high frequencies (up to 20 Hz) are delivered. A high-pressure gas source, fed into a continuous positive airway pressure (CPAP) circuit immediately opposite the endotracheal tube connector, is interrupted. During HFOV, even smaller tidal volumes are delivered at frequencies between 8 and 15 Hz. Various techniques are used to generate HFOV and include a sine wave pump and a diaphragm driven by a linear motor. The delivered volume is inversely related to frequency with all oscillators [8], and hence frequencies between 5 and 10 Hz rather than faster rates can be more effective in infants who have severe carbon dioxide retention. Unlike other forms of respiratory support, HFOV has an active expiratory as well as an active inspiratory phase. Certain oscillators allow an inspiratory/expiratory ratio of up to 1:2 to reduce the likelihood of gas trapping. Use of a 1:2 ratio is associated with lower volume delivery, MAP, and poorer oxygenation) [9], and it has been demonstrated that even under extreme conditions (high resistance and high compliance), gas trapping did not occur with an inspiratory/expiratory ratio of 1:1 [10]. HFOV has been used with either a low-volume strategy in which the MAP is limited with the aim of preventing damage from baro/voluotrauma, or a high-volume strategy in which MAP is elevated to promote optimum alveolar recruitment and expansion and avoid damage from atelectotrauma. Comparisons have only been undertaken in animal models, but the evidence is compelling that the high-volume strategy is less damaging to the lungs [11]. In infants who have severe respiratory failure, transfer to a high-volume HFOV strategy results in increased MAP in an attempt to improve oxygenation. Assessment of lung volume by a helium gas dilution technique before transfer to HFOV can predict the change in MAP necessary to optimize oxygenation [12].

Noninvasive respiratory support

CPAP can be delivered by a headbox, facemask, nasaopharyngeal or endotracheal tubes, single or dual nasal prongs, or a high-flow nasal cannula. Nowadays, the first two methods are rarely used. Studies have demonstrated that the method of CPAP delivery influences outcome. In one randomized trial, use of binasal prongs versus a nasopharyngeal prong was associated with a lower oxygen requirement and respiratory rate [13]. Meta-analysis of the results of two randomized trials evaluating CPAP following extubation demonstrated that short binasal prongs were more effective at preventing re-intubation than a single or nasopharyngeal prong (RR 0.59 (0.41–0.85)) [13].

In another study, however, the CPAP duration was shorter in very low birth weight infants when a nasopharyngeal prong was used rather than binasal prongs [14]. During "bubble" CPAP, the pressure in the device is generated by a continuous flow of gas with the distal end placed a set depth under water. The bubbles create pressure oscillations, which are transmitted back to the airway opening. Lung mechanics and applied flow influence the magnitude of the noise superimposed on the transmitted pressure wave form during bubble CPAP [15]. However, in a randomized crossover trial of 26 infants with a mean gestational age of 27 weeks, vigorous, high-amplitude bubbling compared with slow bubbling CPAP (each examined for 30 minutes) did not result in any significant differences with regard to respiratory rate, pulse oximetry, and transcutaneous carbon dioxide tensions [16].

It has been suggested that the chests of infants who receive bubble CPAP by way of an endotracheal tube vibrate in a similar manner and frequency to those who receive HFOV [17], and as a consequence it was hypothesized that bubble CPAP might reduce the work of breathing and augment gas exchange by facilitated diffusion. Lee and colleagues [17] were subsequently able to demonstrate that despite reduction in minute ventilation and respiratory rate on bubble CPAP compared with ventilator-derived CPAP in intubated infants, blood gas parameters were maintained. Variable flow CPAP is by way of nasal prongs or a modified nasal cannula, and the work of breathing is lower. The positive effects may result from gas entrainment by the high-velocity jet flows. Lung overdistension, however, may occur in infants who have mild disease if variable flow CPAP levels greater than 6 cmH_2O are used.

Although nasal CPAP is considered by many as a gentler form of respiratory support [18], it does have adverse effects including nasal trauma. In some studies, this has been reported to be common; 20% of infants supported on dual prongs were affected in one series [19] and 32% in another [20]. It had been suggested that trauma may particularly be problematic with dual prongs, but randomized studies have demonstrated no significant differences in the incidence of trauma between binasal prongs and nasopharyngeal tube [14], or binasal prongs and facemask [20]. The only significant relationship to trauma in one series was CPAP duration [20].

Continuous negative distending pressure (CNEP) is an alternative way of providing distending pressure. The infant's body is placed in a negative pressure box from which the head protrudes, and CNEP of -4 to -10 cmH_2O is applied [21].

Extracorporeal membrane oxygenation

Extracorporeal membrane oxygenation (ECMO) is a form of cardiopulmonary bypass in which the circulation is diverted from the body and pumped through a silicon membrane oxygenator. Cannulation for ECMO is either venoarterial or venovenous. During venoarterial ECMO, total bypass can be achieved and the level of respiratory support can be reduced to limit further trauma to the lungs. In venovenous ECMO, total cardiopulmonary bypass is not achieved and the infant must have reasonable myocardial function. ECMO has traditionally been used in term or near-term infants to treat reversible respiratory failure, when it is felt that the risk of death exceeds 80% and all other therapies have failed.

Inhaled nitric oxide

Inhaled nitric oxide (iNO), administered directly to the airway, is a selective pulmonary vasodilator used to treat hypoxemic respiratory failure associated with pulmonary hypertension of the newborn. Studies in term infants have demonstrated that levels of 5 ppm are equally as effective as higher doses [22,23]. In addition, four dose–response studies have demonstrated that the maximum beneficial effect is seen at levels of less than 30 ppm, and increases of up to 80 to 100 ppm did not result in further improvements in oxygenation [24]. Side effects are more likely at higher doses. Nitric oxide reacts with oxygen to form nitrogen dioxide (NO_2), and the reaction rate is proportional to the square of the nitric oxide concentration. NO_2 is toxic to the lungs; humans inhaling 2 to 3 ppm for 3 to 5 hours had reductions in antioxidant defenses and an increase in alveolar permeability. In addition, reactive species such as peroxynitrite formed from NO_2 have the potential to damage DNA, raising the possibility of mutagenic or carcinogenic effects. Nitric oxide should only be administered where there is immediate access to methemoglobin analysis. The nitrosylhemoglobin produced by nitric oxide binding to hemoglobin is rapidly converted to methemoglobin, which is then reduced by methemoglobin reductase in the erythrocytes. Premature infants and those of certain ethnic origins have low levels of methemoglobin reductase. It is important, therefore, to assess methemoglobin levels immediately before and during iNO therapy.

Liquid ventilation

Liquid ventilation is performed by filling the lungs with perfluorocarbons (PFC). PFC, compared with water, have a low surface tension and a high solubility for respiratory gases. Liquid ventilation can be applied as total liquid ventilation in which the oxygenated PFC are instilled into the lung and the ventilator circuit is filled with PFC. The PFC are then moved backward and forward from the circuit into the lungs. The alternative technique is partial liquid ventilation, during which the PFC are instilled into the lungs at a volume equivalent to the expected functional residual capacity and the infant's endotracheal tube is connected to a conventional ventilator.

Ventilator/oscillator performance

A square airway pressure wave form is often assumed during IPPV, but ventilators may be unable to maintain such a wave form at fast rates and short inflation times [25]. Certain new neonatal ventilators allow the rise time to peak pressure to be varied. Physiologic data suggest a rapid rather than a slurred upstroke is more likely to provoke active expiration/asynchrony [26]. Asynchrony does occur in the population of premature infants [27]. Whether this is reduced by use of a slurred upstroke to positive pressure inflation has to be appropriately tested. Delivered volume is compromised in certain ventilators when rate is increased or inflation time reduced [28]. Many studies have shown differences in the performance of different types of triggering systems. The most compelling evidence is from a study [29] in which two different triggering systems were assessed using a single neonatal ventilator, thus any difference noted was from the triggering system and not the ventilator. This study demonstrated that pressure triggering compared with airflow triggering had a lower sensitivity and a longer trigger delay (also referred to as *response time*), which could translate into a higher air leak rate. In VTV, there are differences according to ventilator type in the delivered peak pressure, inflation time, and MAP. These related to differences in the airway pressure wave forms delivered by the different ventilator types: airway pressure wave forms vary from a square wave form with a positive pressure plateau; termination of the peak pressure once the preset volume has been delivered (decelerating wave form); and a slurred upstroke in the inflating pressure, with the delivered volume only being achieved at the end of the preset inflation time [30]. Various techniques have been used to generate HFOV and this influences the airway pressure wave form and the volume delivered [31]. Despite using the same oscillatory settings, volumes vary according to oscillator type, but, as the frequency is increased, the volume delivered falls with all oscillators [8].

Monitoring

The newer generation of ventilators displays the delivered volume and thus it is tempting to use these values to determine the most appropriate level of volume delivery. Physiologic studies, however, have demonstrated that the delivered volume may vary considerably even when infants have blood gases within the "therapeutic" range, because their spontaneous respiratory efforts may make a sizeable contribution to minute ventilation [32]. In addition, the monitors may be inaccurate. For example, in a physiologic study examining the VIP BIRD ventilator, the actual volume delivery was always significantly higher than the volume displayed by the ventilator and incidentally lower than the preset level [30]. The latter difference results from compressible volume loss in the circuit and is also influenced by gas leaks around the uncuffed endotracheal tubes used in neonates. Frequency can affect the accuracy of the volumes displayed by oscillators [33]. Comparison of the displayed versus the measured volumes using a lung model and a sine wave pump (which delivered a constant volume) demonstrated that the SLE 5000 overread by 5%, but at 5 Hz the Draeger 8000 Plus and Stephanie ventilators underread by 20%. Increasing the frequency from 5 to 15 Hz resulted in even greater discrepancy between the measured and displayed volumes by the Stephanie oscillator. It is important then to check arterial blood gases soon after changing frequency rather than rely on the oscillator volume display, particularly because abrupt reductions in carbon dioxide tension during HFOV can cause large changes in cerebral blood flow velocity [34].

Acute respiratory distress in preterm infants

Time-cycled, pressure-limited ventilation

IPPV has been the most frequently used mode for the newborn. Meta-analysis of the results of randomized trials demonstrated the risk for air leaks was lower with HFPPV compared with slower rate IPPV (RR 0.69, 95% CI 0.51,0.93) [35]. Faster rates reduce active expiration [2] and hence may have reduced the risk of pneumothorax. The trials, however, were performed before the routine use of antenatal corticosteroids and postnatal surfactant. Whether HFPPV compared with slow rate IPPV reduces the risk of pneumothoraces in the present population of prematurely born infants has not been appropriately tested.

Patient-triggered ventilation

Physiologic studies demonstrated benefits for either A/C or SIMV, including less asynchrony, reduced cerebral blood flow fluctuations, and lower work of breathing, but the comparator was often intermittent mandatory ventilation. No significant differences in the rates of bronchopulmonary dysplasia (BPD), severe intracranial hemorrhage (ICH), air leaks, and mortality according to ventilation mode, however, were demonstrated in the meta-analysis [35] of the results of randomized trials. Although the meta-analysis did not demonstrate any significant excess of adverse effects [35], in the largest trial [36] included in the meta-analysis, there was a trend for more immature infants supported by A/C to have air leaks. It is possible that the results of the A/C arm of the trial were adversely affected by using an airway pressure trigger in most infants on A/C [29]. The meta-analysis, however, did demonstrate that patient-triggered ventilation was associated with a shorter duration of ventilation, but this was only seen in infants recovering from rather than in the acute stages of respiratory distress [37]. In three trials, A/C has been compared with weaning by SIMV in infants recovering from respiratory distress syndrome (RDS)

[38,39]. In all three trials, the infants were supported by a single ventilator type, and weaning in the A/C arm was by pressure reduction only. The method of weaning by SIMV, however, differed. In one trial, during SIMV the peak inflating pressure was reduced and the rate decreased to 5 bpm before extubation—this resulted in a significantly longer duration of weaning. In the trial in which the SIMV rate was decreased to a minimum of 20 bpm, the duration of weaning by SIMV and A/C was similar. In these trials, spontaneous breaths were supported solely by PEEP [38,39], and the likely explanation for the difference in the results of the trials is that reduction in the number of breaths supported by mechanical inflations below 20 per minute increases the work of breathing related to overcoming the imposed work of breathing. In support of that hypothesis, oxygen consumption has increased at low ventilator rates [40]. SIMV has also been an inferior weaning mode in randomized trials in adults. PSV has been associated with a lower rate of asynchrony [41] and thus might reduce air leaks, but this has not yet been tested in a randomized trial. In a short-term study, PAV allowed adequate gas exchange at lower MAPs than A/C and IMV in premature infants [42] and was associated with a lower incidence of thoracoabdominal asynchrony and chest wall distortion than CPAP [43].

Volume-targeted ventilation

Meta-analysis of the results of four randomized trials [4] demonstrated VTV was associated with significant reductions in the duration of ventilation and the rate of pneumothorax, but not death or BPD. The trials, however, were small, including a total 178 infants. In two studies, volume-controlled ventilation was examined and in the other two VG was studied. In addition, the design of the two volume-controlled ventilation trials limits the generalizability of their results. In one [44], IPPV was not delivered by a comparable neonatal ventilator, and in the second [45], the airway pressure wave form on the IPPV mode differed from that delivered by other neonatal ventilators in that there was no positive pressure plateau [46]. A further randomized trial comparing volume-controlled ventilation to time-cycled, pressure-limited ventilation using the VIP BIRD has recently been published [47]. Among infants weighing between 600 and 1500 g and gestational ages 24 to 31 weeks and have RDS, those on volume-controlled ventilation reached predetermined success criteria faster; the difference reached statistical significance in babies weighing less than 1000 g. There were, however, no significant differences in the duration of ventilation or occurrence of complications. However, all respiratory-related deaths in the first week of life occurred exclusively in the IPPV group. During VG, adequate gas exchange is achieved at lower MAPs [48], because the baby makes a greater contribution to minute ventilation [41]. Results of randomized trials have suggested that addition of VG to A/C allows more rapid improvement in oxygenation, particularly in infants who have a birth weight of less than 1000 g [48]. In another randomized study, a VG level of 4 mL/kg with SIMV rather than SIMV alone was more effective with regard to maintaining desirable carbon dioxide tensions in infants greater than 25 weeks of gestational age, but was ineffective in more immature infants [49]. Volume targeting may be more effective when used with A/C rather than SIMV, as evidenced by a lower work of breathing [50].

Whether the use of VG in combination with PSV improves outcomes remains controversial, particularly with regard to the effect on lung inflammation [51,52]. In one study, the only advantage of using VG with PSV was less blood gas monitoring [53], but in another, the MAP was higher than during SIMV without VG [54].

High-frequency ventilation

In one randomized study, use of HFJV was associated with a reduction in the incidence of BPD at 36 weeks and less need for home oxygen [55], but a second trial [56] was halted for safety reasons, because infants exposed to HFJV had higher rates of severe ICH (41% versus 22%) and periventricular leukomalacia (PVL) (31% versus 6%). There have been at least 11 trials in which infants have been randomized to receive HFOV or standard ventilation techniques in the first 24 hours after birth. Meta-analysis of their results [57] demonstrated that HFOV had no significant effect on mortality, only a modest reduction in BPD in survivors at term, but no statistically significant effect on short-term neurologic abnormality, ICH, or PVL. The 3 most recently reported randomized trials included in the meta-analysis yielded different results. Moriette and colleagues [58] reported that HFOV was associated with a trend toward an increase in severe ICH; the type of oscillator used in their trial has not been used in any of the other randomized studies. Courtney and colleagues [59] reported that HFOV reduced the combined outcome of BPD and death, but the randomized comparator group was supported solely by SIMV, which may have put them at a disadvantage because the work of breathing is increased at low SIMV rates [40]. In the third trial [31] (United Kingdom Oscillation, UKOS trial), 799 infants below 29 weeks of gestation were randomized within 1 hour of birth to HFOV or standard ventilation techniques, and no benefits or disadvantages of HFOV were noted. In addition, the follow-up assessments of the UKOS survivors also demonstrated no significant differences in the results of lung function measurements at 1 year of age [60] or respiratory or neurodevelopmental outcome at 2 years of corrected age [61].

Noninvasive respiratory support

CPAP is now used in many centers in preference to early intubation and IPPV [18,62–64]. In nonrandomized trials, its use has been associated with a reduction in the requirement for mechanical ventilation and the incidence of BPD. Yet, meta-analysis of two published randomized trials examining whether prophylactic CPAP commenced soon after birth reduced the use of mechanical ventilation, and the incidence of BPD demonstrated no significant differences in any of the outcomes [65]. In addition, in a randomized study including 230 infants of gestational ages 29 to 31 weeks, prophylactic CPAP (instituted within 30 minutes of birth) was not found more efficacious than rescue CPAP, applied when the inspired oxygen requirement was greater than 40%, with regard to need for surfactant treatment or mechanical ventilation [66]. In another randomized study [67], however, infants who developed RDS and were given surfactant and subsequently randomized to immediate extubation and nasal CPAP required a shorter duration of oxygen therapy, nasal CPAP, and mechanical ventilation than those randomized to remain on mechanical ventilation. Meta-analysis of the results of postextubation randomized trials has demonstrated that CPAP significantly reduced the need for additional respiratory support [RR 0.62 (0.49–0.77)], but not the need for endotracheal intubation [RR 0.93 (0.72–1.19)] or supplemental oxygen requirement at 28 days [RR 1.00 (0.81–1.24)] [68].

The evidence for benefit of nasal ventilation modes, including IPPV, SIMV, or HFOV delivered by nasal prongs is from either anecdotal studies or from trials with only short-term outcomes, and it remains uncertain whether they have significant adverse outcomes [69–71]. Randomized trials comparing nasal IPPV with CPAP in infants who have apnea of prematurity have yielded conflicting results. One trial [72] showed no differences, whereas the other [73] concluded that nasal IPPV was associated with a reduction in apnea frequency. Meta-analysis of the results of the two trials demonstrated no significant differences in carbon dioxide elimination at the end of the 4- to 6-hour study period.

Early studies [74] demonstrated CNEP was associated with improvements in oxygenation in infants who have severe RDS. In a randomized trial [75], use of CNEP (-4 to–6 cmH$_2$O) was associated with a lower duration of oxygen therapy (18.3 versus 33.6 days), but there were trends toward increases in mortality and cranial ultrasound abnormalities in the CNEP group.

Severe lung disease

High-frequency oscillatory ventilation

There have been two randomized trials of HFOV in infants who have severe respiratory failure. In term infants [76], although HFOV was a more effective rescue therapy than IPPV, there were no significant differences in the requirement for ECMO or duration of ventilator or oxygen dependency between the two groups. In preterm infants, use of HFOV was associated with a significant reduction in new pulmonary air leaks (RR 0.73, 95% CI 0.55–0.96), but a significant increase in ICH (RR 1.77, 95% CI 1.06–2.96) [77]. High-volume strategy HFOV is not a successful form of rescue support in all babies who have severe respiratory disease, and failure to improve oxygenation after 6 hours of a high-volume strategy identifies those babies most likely to die [78] or survive with disability [79]. An initial improvement in oxygenation in response to HFOV, however, does not guarantee a normal neurodevelopmental outcome at 2 years in prematurely born infants [80].

Extracorporeal membrane oxygenation

Two early trials performed in the United States using adaptive experimental designs demonstrated the efficacy of neonatal ECMO in severe respiratory failure. In a multicenter United Kingdom randomized trial of 185 infants who had an oxygenation index greater than 40, ECMO compared with conventional ventilation was associated with a 50% reduction in mortality in infants who had persistent pulmonary hypertension of the newborn (PPHN) or meconium aspiration syndrome (MAS). The ELSO data highlight that ECMO survival figures vary according to diagnosis with survival rates of 90% for infants who have MAS, 76% for larger infants who have RDS, and only 50% for infants who have congenital diaphragmatic hernia (CDH).

Inhaled nitric oxide

Meta-analysis of the results of randomized trials has demonstrated that iNO reduces the need for ECMO or death in infants born at or near term, but the positive effect is on ECMO requirement [81]. Meta-analysis [82] of the results of seven trials in premature infants demonstrated that iNO had short-term positive effects on oxygenation, but no significant effects on mortality, BPD, or ICH. In one study [83], however, iNO was associated with a significant reduction in the combined outcome of death and BPD (RR 0.76, 0.60–0.97) and in grade 3 and 4 IVH (RR 0.51, 0.27–0.97); subanalysis demonstrated the advantages were seen in the infants who had mild disease. In contrast, in infants who had severe respiratory failure, the use of iNO was associated with prolongation of intensive care and increased cost of care without clear beneficial effects [84]. Recently, two positive iNO studies have been reported; both suggest that prolonged therapy with iNO may be more efficacious. In one [85], although overall there was no reduction in death or BPD, in infants with birth weights between 1000 and 1250 g, low-dose (5 ppm) iNO reduced the incidence of BPD by 50% and in this cohort was associated with a lower rate of the combined outcome of ICH, PVL, and ventriculomegaly. In that trial, iNO was given for 21 days or until extubation. In the second trial [86], iNO was associated with a significant increase in survival without BPD (43.9% versus 36.8%); the minimum treatment exposure was 24 days. The infants who received iNO were discharged sooner and received supplemental oxygen for a shorter time. Posthoc analysis demonstrated that the positive effects were seen in infants enrolled at 7 to 14 days but not at 15 to 21 days and were restricted to infants who had less-severe lung disease.

Liquid ventilation

There are limited data on liquid ventilation. In a nonrandomized, un-blinded study, premature infants who had severe RDS in whom conventional ventilation had failed were treated with partial liquid ventilation for up to 96 hours; they experienced significant increases in their arterial oxygen tension and dynamic compliance [87]. Similarly, dynamic pulmonary compliance significantly increased [88] in response to partial liquid ventilation in six term infants who had respiratory failure who showed no improvement while receiving ECMO.

Pulmonary interstitial emphysema

Increasing the ventilator rate to 100 to 120 bpm on conventional ventilation can reduce the number of infants who have pulmonary interstitial emphysema (PIE) who develop pneumothorax, but the severity of their PIE worsens [89]. Oxygenation in infants who have severe PIE has been reported in small nonrandomized series to improve when continuous negative pressure is combined with intermittent mandatory ventilation or infants are transferred from conventional ventilation to HFOV or HFJV. In randomized trials, however, high-frequency oscillatory was not of greater benefit than positive pressure ventilation [77], but HFJV use was associated with more rapid resolution of PIE [90]. HFFI use has also been associated with improvements in blood gases in babies who have PIE and radiologic resolution of the PIE [91], but only in anecdotal studies.

Meconium aspiration syndrome

Oxygenation of infants who have severe MAS may improve if HFJV is used in combination with surfactant [92]. Similarly, HFOV has improved oxygenation in infants who have severe MAS; the combination of HFOV and iNO may be particularly efficacious [93]. The most compelling evidence is from a randomized trial in which ECMO improved the survival of infants who had MAS with an oxygenation index greater than 40 by 50% [94]. Data from the ELSO registry highlight that approximately 94% of infants who have MAS placed on ECMO survive, and other results suggest that this is not associated with an increased risk of neurologic disability.

Pulmonary hypertension

In uncontrolled studies, hyperventilation to achieve carbon dioxide tensions of 20 to 25 torr and an elevation of pH resulted in improvements in oxygenation [95], but such low CO_2 levels are associated with a 50% reduction in cerebral blood flow, and hypocarbia has been associated with PVL in preterm infants [96]. Moreover, the technique of hyperventilation was described for primary pulmonary hypertension of the newborn, whereby the pathophysiology was increased pulmonary vascular resistance in the absence of pulmonary parenchymal disease. Applying this technique to parenchymal lung diseases, especially MAS, may be dangerous. Even in the early studies, hyperventilation was associated with an increase in air leak and BPD [97]. Both HFJV and HFOV anecdotally have improved oxygenation in infants who have pulmonary hypertension, but no long-term benefits have been investigated. In contrast, in a randomized trial, ECMO improved survival in infants who have severe PPHN [95].

Congenital diaphragmatic hernia

Preoperative stabilization of infants who have CDH reduces mortality [98,99]. Refractory hypoxemia on conventional ventilation anecdotally responds to HFJV and HFOV, but there are no proven long-term benefits of either. Although ECMO is frequently considered for infants who have CDH, in a randomized trial no benefit in survival was associated with ECMO use [96]. Inhaled nitric oxide does not reduce the need for ECMO in infants who have CDH [100].

Bronchopulmonary dysplasia

A major aim of respiratory support for babies who have established BPD is to minimize further trauma to the lungs. Conventional ventilator techniques have been studied in infants developing BPD. Rates over 60 bpm have not been demonstrated to offer advantages over lower rates [101], but increasing the PEEP to 6 cmH_2O can improve oxygenation without adversely affecting carbon dioxide elimination [102]. Patient-triggered ventilation and HFOV have been used with short-term success in infants who have BPD, but the evidence is anecdotal. Some studies have examined the efficacy of iNO in infants who have BPD. In infants who have early BPD, a level of 20 ppm was associated with improvements in oxygenation without inducing changes in inflammatory markers or oxidative injury [103]. In a nonrandomized study of BPD infants [104], a positive rather than no response was associated with a better long-term outcome; those who responded were ultimately weaned from the ventilator, whereas the five nonresponders died or failed to be weaned.

Summary

The early days of mechanical ventilation of newborns who have respiratory failure were limited to few ventilator types and established techniques, leading to a uniform approach no matter what the specific cause of the respiratory failure. Our understanding of neonatal pulmonary pathophysiology has increased dramatically over the past 25 years, as has the technology now available to treat it. Recent clinical trials clearly demonstrate the value of different approaches to different diseases, but the evidence base must be expanded if better long-term outcomes are to be achieved.

References

[1] Greenough A, Pool J, Greenall F, et al. Comparison of different rates of artificial ventilation in preterm neonates with the respiratory distress syndrome. Acta Paediatr Scand 1987; 76:706–12.

[2] Greenough A, Greenall F, Gamsu H. Synchronous respiration–which ventilator rate is best? Acta Paediatr Scand 1987;76:713–8.

[3] Schulze A, Schaller P. Proportional assist ventilation: a new strategy for infant ventilation? Neonatal Respir Dis 1996;6:1–10.

[4] McCallion N, Davis PG, Morley CJ. Volume targeted versus pressure limited ventilation in the neonate. Cochrane Database Syst Rev 2005;3:CD003666.

[5] Dawson C, Davies MW. Volume-targeted ventilation and arterial carbon dioxide in neonates. J Paediatr Child Health 2005;41:518–21.

[6] Polimeni V, Claure N, D'Ugard C, et al. Effects of volume-targeted synchronized intermittent mandatory ventilation on spontaneous episodes of hypoxemia in preterm infants. Biol Neonate 2006;89(1):50–5.

[7] Sharma A, Rafferty G, Milner A, et al. Volume guarantee level and work of breathing during neonatal ventilation. Eur Respir J 2006;28(Suppl 50):P2833.

[8] Laubscher B, Greenough A, Costeloe K. Performance of four neonatal high frequency oscillators. British Journal of Intensive Care 1996;6:148–52.

[9] Dimitriou G, Greenough A, Kavvadia V, et al. Comparison of two inspiratory expiratory ratios during high frequency oscillation. Eur J Pediatr 1999;158:796–9.

[10] Leipala J, Milner AD, Greenough A. An in vitro assessment of gas trapping during high frequency oscillation. Physiol Meas 2005;26:329–36.

[11] McCulloch PR, Fokert PG, Froese AB. Lung volume maintenance prevents lung injury during high frequency oscillatory ventilation in surfactant deficient rabbits. Am Rev Respir Dis 1988;137:1185–92.

[12] Dimitriou G, Cheeseman P, Greenough A. Lung volume and the response to high volume strategy, high frequency oscillation. Acta Paediatr 2004;93(5):613–7.

[13] De Paoli AG, Davis PG, Faber B, et al. Devices and pressure sources for administration of nasal continuous positive airway pressure (NCPAP) in preterm neonates. Cochrane Database Syst Rev 2002;4:CD002977.

[14] Buettiker V, Hug MI, Baenziger O, et al. Advantages and disadvantages of different nasal CPAP systems in newborns. Intensive Care Med 2004;30:926–30.

[15] Pillow J, Travadi JN, Bubble CPAP. Is the noise important? An in vitro study. Pediatr Res 2005;57:826–30.

[16] Morley CJ, Lau R, De Paoli A, et al. Nasal continuous positive airway pressure: does bubbling improve gas exchange. Arch Dis Child Fetal Neonatal Ed 2005;90:343–4.

[17] Lee KS, Dunn MS, Fenwick M, et al. A comparison of underwater bubble continuous positive airway pressure with ventilator-derived continuous positive airway pressure in premature neonates ready for extubation. Biol Neonate 1998;73(2):69–75.

[18] Jacobsen T, Gronvall J, Petersen S, et al. "Minitouch" treatment of very low-birth-weight infants. Acta Paed 1993;82:934–8.

[19] Robertson NJ, McCarthy LS, Hamilton PA, et al. Nasal deformities resulting from flow driver continuous positive airway pressure. Arch Dis Child Fetal Neonatal Ed 1996; 75(3):F209–12.

[20] Yong SC, Chen SJ, Boo NY. Incidence of nasal trauma associated with nasal prong versus nasal mask during continuous positive airway pressure treatment in very low birthweight infants: a randomised control study. Arch Dis Child Fetal Neonatal Ed 2005;90:F480–3.

[21] Samuels MP, Southall DP. Negative extrathoracic pressure in neonatal respiratory failure. Pediatrics 1989;98:1154–60.

[22] Davidson D, Barefield ES, Kattwinkel J, et al. Inhaled nitric oxide for the early treatment of persistent pulmonary hypertension of the newborn: a randomized, double-masked, placebo-controlled, dose reponse, multicenter study. Pediatrics 1998;101:325–34.

[23] Wood KS, McCaffery MJ, Donovan JC, et al. Effect of initial nitric oxide concentration on outcome in infants with pulmonary hypertension. Biol Neonate 1999;75:215–24.

[24] Macrae DJ, Field D, Mercier JC, et al. Inhaled nitric oxide therapy in neonates and children: reaching a European consensus. Intensive Care Med 2004;30(3):372–80.

[25] Greenough A, Greenall F. Performance of respirators at fast rates commonly used in the neonatal intensive care unit. Pediatr Pulmonol 1987;3:357–61.

[26] Greenough A. The premature infant's respiratory response to mechanical ventilation. Early Hum Dev 1988;17:1–5.

[27] Sharma A, Rafferty G, Milner AD, et al. Interaction of spontaneous respiration with conventional and triggered ventilation. Eur Respir J 2006;28(Suppl 50):P2830.

[28] Dimitriou G, Greenough A. Performance of neonatal ventilators. British Journal of Intensive Care 2000;10:186–8.

[29] Dimitriou G, Greenough A, Cherian S. Comparison of airway pressure and air flow triggering systems using a single type of neonatal ventilator. Acta Paediatr 2001;90:445–7.

[30] Sharma A, Sylvester K, Milner AD, et al. Performance of neonatal ventilators in volume guarantee mode. Acta Paediatrica, in press.

[31] Johnson AH, Peacock JL, Greenough A, et al. For the United Kingdom Oscillation Study Group. High frequency oscillatory ventilation for the prevention of chronic lung disease of prematurity. N Engl J Med 2002;347:633–42.

[32] Sharma A, Rafferty G, Milner AD, et al. Determination of appropriate volume delivery during neonatal volume targeted ventilation. Eur Respir J 2006;28(Suppl 50):P2828.

[33] Leipala J, Iwasaki S, Milner AD, et al. Accuracy of the volume and pressure displays of high frequency oscillators. Arch Dis Child Fetal Neonatal Ed 2004;24:731–3.

[34] Kavvadia V, Greenough A, Boylan G, et al. Effect of a high volume strategy high frequency oscillation on cerebral haemodynamics. Eur J Pediatr 2001;160:140–1.

[35] Greenough A, Milner AD, Dimitriou G. Synchronized ventilation. Cochrane Database Syst Rev 2005;3:CD000456.

[36] Baumer JH. International randomized controlled trial of patient triggered ventilation in neonatal respiratory distress syndrome. Arch Dis Child Fetal Neonatal Ed 2000;82:F5–10.

[37] Chan V, Greenough A. Randomised controlled trial of weaning by patient triggered ventilation or conventional ventilation. Eur J Pediatr 1993;152:51–4.

[38] Chan V, Greenough A. Comparison of weaning by patient triggered ventilation or synchronous intermittent mandatory ventilation in preterm infants. Acta Paediatr 1994;83:335–7.

[39] Dimitriou G, Greenough A, Giffin F, et al. Synchronous intermittent mandatory ventilation modes compared with patient triggered ventilation during weaning. Arch Dis Child Fetal Neonatal Ed 1995;72:F188–90.

[40] Roze JC, Liet JM, Gournay V, et al. Oxygen cost of breathing and weaning process in newborn infants. Eur Respir J 1997;10:2583–5.

[41] Dimitriou G, Greenough A, Laubscher B, et al. Comparison of airway pressure triggered and airflow triggered ventilation in very immature infants. Acta Paediatr 1998;87:1256–60.

[42] Schulze A, Gerhardt T, Musante G, et al. Proportional assist ventilation in low birthweight infants with acute respiratory disease: a comparison to assist/control and conventional mechanical ventilation. J Pediatr 1999;135:339–44.

[43] Musante G, Schulze A, Gerhardt T, et al. Proportional assist ventilation decreases thoracoabdominal asynchrony and chest wall distortion in preterm infants. Pediatr Res 2001;49:175–80.

[44] Piotrowski A, Sobala W, Kawczynski P. Patient-initiated, pressure-regulated, volume-controlled ventilation compared with intermittent mandatory ventilation in neonates: a prospective, randomized study. Intensive Care Med 1997;23:975–81.

[45] Sinha SK, Donn SM, Gavey J, et al. Randomized trial of volume controlled versus time cycled, pressure limited ventilation in preterm infants with respiratory distress syndrome. Arch Dis Child Fetal Neonatal Ed 1997;77:F202–5.

[46] Greenough A, Milner A, Dimitriou G. Volume controlled and time cycled pressure limited ventilation. Arch Dis Child Fetal Neonatal Ed 1998;79:F79–80.

[47] Singh J, Sinha SK, Clarke P, et al. Mechanical ventilation of very low birth weight infants: is volume or pressure a better target variable? J Pediatr 2006;149(3):308–13.

[48] Cheema IU, Ahluwalia JS. Feasibility of tidal volume-guided ventilation in newborn infants: a randomized, cross over trial using the volume guarantee modality. Pediatrics 2001;107:1323–8.

[49] Cheema IU, Sinha AK, Kempley ST, et al. Impact of volume guarantee ventilation on arterial carbon dioxide tension in newborn infants: a randomized controlled trial. Early Hum Dev 2006; in press.

[50] Abubakar KM, Keszler M. Patient-ventilator interactions in new modes of patient triggered ventilation. Pediatr Pulmonol 2001;32(1):71–5.

[51] Lista G, Colnaghi M, Castolidi F, et al. Impact of targeted volume ventilation on lung inflammatory response in preterm infants with respiratory distress syndrome (RDS). Pediatr Pulmonol 2004;37:510–4.

[52] Dani C, Bertini G, Pezzati M, et al. Effects of pressure support ventilation plus volume guarantee vs. high-frequency oscillatory ventilation on lung inflammation in preterm infants. Pediatr Pulmonol 2006;41(3):242–9.

[53] Nafday SM, Green RS, Lin J, et al. Is there an advantage of using pressure support ventilation with volume guarantee in the initial management of premature infants with respiratory distress syndrome? A pilot study. J Perinatol 2005;25:193–7.

[54] Olsen SL, Thibeault DW, Truog WE. Crossover trial comparing pressure support with synchronized intermittent mandatory ventilation. J Perinatol 2002;22:461–6.

[55] Keszler M, Modanlou HD, Brudno S, et al. Multicentre controlled clinical trial of high frequency jet ventilation in preterm infants with uncomplicated respiratory distress syndrome. Pediatrics 1997;100(4):593–9.

[56] Wiswell TE, Graziani LJ, Kornhauser MS, et al. High frequency jet ventilation in the early management of respiratory distress syndrome is associated with a greater risk for adverse outcomes. Pediatrics 1996;98:1035–43.

[57] Henderson-Smart DJ, Bhuta T, Cools F, et al. Elective high frequency oscillatory ventilation versus conventional ventilation for acute pulmonary dysfunction in preterm infants. Cochrane Syst Rev 2005;3:CD000104.

[58] Moriette G, Paris-Llado J, Walti H, et al. Prospective randomized multicentre comparison of high frequency oscillatory ventilation and conventional ventilation in preterm infants less than 30 weeks with respiratory distress syndrome. Pediatrics 2001;107: 363–72.

[59] Courtney SE, Durand DJ, Asselin JM, et al. Neonatal Ventilation Study Group. High frequency oscillatory ventilation versus conventional mechanical ventilation for very low birthweight infants. N Engl J Med 2002;347:643–52.

[60] Thomas M, Rafferty G, Limb E, et al. Pulmonary function at follow-up of very preterm infants form the UK oscillation study. Am J Respir Crit Care Med 2004;169:868–72.

[61] Marlow N, Peacock J, Greenough A, et al. Randomised trial of high frequency oscillatory ventilation or conventional ventilation in babies of 28 weeks or less gestational age: respiratory and neurological outcomes at two years. Arch Dis Child Fetal Neonatal Ed 2006; 91(5):F320–6.

[62] Avery ME, Tooley WH, Keller JB, et al. Is chronic lung disease in low birthweight infants preventable? A survey of eight centers. Pediatrics 1987;79:26–30.

[63] Kamper J, Wulff K, Larsen C, et al. Early treatment with nasal continuous positive pressure in very low birthweight infants. Acta Pediatrics 1993;88:880–4.

[64] Verder H, Robertson B, Griesen G, et al. Surfactant therapy and nasal continuous positive airways pressure for newborns with respiratory distress syndrome. N Engl J Med 1994;331: 1051–5.

[65] Subramaniam P, Henderson-Smart D, Davis PJ. Prophylactic nasal continuous positive airway pressure for preventing morbidity and mortality in very preterm infants. Cochrane Database Syst Rev 2005;3:CD001243.

[66] Sandri F, Ancora G, Lanzoni A, et al. Prophylactic nasal continuous positive airways pressure in newborns of 28-31 weeks gestation: multicentre randomized controlled trial. Arch Dis Child 2004;89:394–8.

[67] Dani C, Bertini G, Pezzati M, et al. Early extubation and nasal continuous positive airway pressure after surfactant treatment for respiratory distress syndrome among preterm infants < 30 weeks gestation. Pediatrics 2004;113:560–3.

[68] Davis PG, Henderson-Smart DJ. Nasal continuous positive airways pressure immediately after exbutation for preventing morbidity in preterm infants. Cochrane Database Syst Rev 2006;3.

[69] Lemyre B, Davis PG, De Paoli AG. Nasal intermittent positive pressure ventilation (NIPPV) versus nasal continuous positive airway pressure (NCPAP) for apnea of prematurity. Cochrane Database Syst Rev 2005;3.

[70] Friedlich P, Lecart C, Posen R, et al. A randomized trial of nasopharyngeal synchronized intermittent mandatory ventilation versus nasopharyngeal continuous positive airway pressure in very low birthweight infants after extubation. J Perinatol 1999;19:413–8.

[71] Van der Hoeven M, Brouwer E, Blanco CE. Nasal high frequency ventilation in neonates with moderate respiratory insufficiency. Arch Dis Child Fetal Neonatal Ed 1998;79:F61–3.

[72] Ryan CA, Finer NN, Peters KL. Nasal intermittent positive-pressure ventilation offers no advantages over nasal continuous positive airway pressure in apnea of prematurity. Am J Dis Child 1989;143(10):1196–8.

[73] Lin CH, Wang ST, Lin YJ, et al. Efficacy of nasal intermittent positive pressure ventilation in treating apnea of prematurity. Pediatr Pulmonol 1998;26(5):349–53.

[74] Outerbridge E. The negative pressure ventilator. In: Thibeault GW, Gregory A, editors. Neonatal pulmonary care. Menlo Park (CA): Addison-Wesley; 1979. p. 168–77.

[75] Samuels MP, Raine J, Wright T, et al. Continuous negative extrathoracic pressure in neonatal respiratory failure. Pediatrics 1996;98:1154–60.

[76] Clark RH, Yoder BA, Sell MS. Prospective, randomized comparison of high frequency oscillation and conventional ventilation in candidates for extracorporeal membrane oxygenation. J Pediatr 1994;124:447–54.

[77] HIFO Study Group. Randomized study of high-frequency oscillatory ventilation in infants with severe respiratory distress. J Pediatr 1993;122:609–19.

[78] Chan V, Greenough A, Gamsu HR. High frequency oscillation for preterm infants with severe respiratory failure. Arch Dis Child Fetal Neonatal Ed 1994;70:F44–6.

[79] Cheung PY, Prasertsom W, Finer NN, et al. Rescue high frequency oscillatory ventilation for preterm infants: neurodevelopmental outcome and its prediction. Biol Neonate 1997;71: 282–91.

[80] Dimitriou G, Greenough A, Broomfield D, et al. Rescue high frequency oscillation, hypocarbia and neurodevelopmental outcome in preterm infants. Early Hum Dev 2002; 66:133–41.

[81] Finer NN, Barrington KJ. Nitric oxide for respiratory failure in infants born at or near term. Cochrane Database Syst Rev 2005;3:CD000399.

[82] Barrington KJ, Finer NN. Inhaled nitric oxide for respiratory failure in preterm infants. Cochrane Database Syst Rev 2006;3.

[83] Schreiber MD, Gin-Mestan K, Marks JD, et al. Inhaled nitric oxide in premature infants with the respiratory distress syndrome. N Engl J Med 2003;349:2099–107.

[84] Field D, Elbourne A, Truesdale R, et al, On behalf of the INNOVO Trial Collaborating Group. Neonatal ventilation with inhaled nitric oxide versus ventilatory support without inhaled nitric oxide for preterm infants with severe respiratory failure. Pedaitrcs 2005; 115:926–36.

[85] Kinsella JP, Cutter GR, Walsh WF, et al. Early inhaled nitric oxide therapy in premature newborns with respiratory failure. N Engl J Med 2006;355:354–64.

[86] Ballard RA, Truog WE, Cnaan A, et al. Inhaled nitric oxide in preterm infants undergoing mechanical ventilation. N Engl J Med 2006;355:343–53.

[87] Leach CL, Greenspan J, Rubenstein SD, et al. Partial liquid ventilation with perfluorocarbon in premature infants with severe respiratory distress syndrome. N Engl J Med 1996;335:761–7.

[88] Greenspan JS, Wolfson M, Holt WJ, et al. Partial liquid ventilation of human preterm neonates. J Pediatr 1997;117:106–11.

[89] Greenough A, Dixon A, Roberton NRC. Pulmonary interstitial emphysema. Arch Dis Child 1984;59:1046–51.

[90] Keszler M, Donn SM, Bucciarelli RL, et al. Multicentre controlled trial comparing high frequency jet ventilation and conventional ventilation in patients with pulmonary interstitial emphysema. J Pediatr 1991;119:85–93.

[91] Davis JM, Richter SE, Kendig JW, et al. High frequency jet ventilation and surfactant treatment of newborns with severe respiratory failure. Pediatr Pulmonol 1992;13:108–12.

[92] Gaylord MS, Quiselll BJ, Lair ME. High frequency ventilation in the treatment of infants weighing less than 1500 gms with pulmonary interstitial emphysema. Pediatrics 1987;79: 915–21.

[93] Kinsella JP, Truog WE, Walsh WF, et al. Randomised multicentre trial of inhaled nitric oxide and high frequency oscillatory ventilation in severe persistent pulmonary hypertension of the newborn. J Pediatr 1997;131(1):55–62.

[94] UK Collaborative ECMO Trial Group. UK collaborative randomised trial of neonatal extracorporeal membrane oxygenation. Lancet 1996;348:75–82.

[95] Peckham GJ, Fox WW. Physiologic factors affecting pulmonary artery pressure in infants with persistent pulmonary hypertension. J Pediatr 1978;93:1005–10.

[96] Greisen G, Munck H, Lou H. Severe hypocarbia in preterm infants with neurodevelopmental deficit. Acta Paediatr Scand 1987;76:401–4.

[97] Beck R. Chronic lung disease following hypocapnic alkalosis for persistent pulmonary hypertension. J Pediatr 1985;106:527–8.

[98] Nio M, Haase G, Kennaugh J, et al. A prospective randomised trial of delayed versus immediate repair of congenital diaphragmatic hernia. J Pediatr Surg 1994;29:618–21.

[99] Cartlidge PH, Mann NP, Kapila A. Preoperative stabilisation in congenital diaphragmatic hernia. Arch Dis Child 1986;61:1226–8.

[100] Finer NN, Barrington KJ. Nitric oxide for respiratory failure in infants born at or near term. Cochrane Database Syst Rev 2001;4:CD000399.

[101] Chan V, Greenough A, Hird MF. Comparison of different rates of artificial ventilation for preterm infants ventilated beyond the first week of life. Early Hum Dev 1991;26:177–83.

[102] Greenough A, Chan V, Hird MF. Positive end expiratory pressure in acute and chronic neonatal respiratory distress. Arch Dis Child 1992;67:320–3.

[103] Clarke PL, Ekekezie IL, Kaftan HA, et al. Safety and efficacy of nitric oxide in chronic lung disease. Arch Dis Child Fetal Neonatal Ed 2002;86:F41–5.

[104] Banks BA, Seri I, Ischiropoulos H, et al. Changes in oxygenation with inhaled nitric oxide in severe bronchopulmonary dysplasia. Pediatrics 1999;103:610–8.

Clin Perinatol 34 (2007) 55–71

The Dreaded Desaturating Baby: A Difficult Problem in Clinical Management

Alan R. Spitzer, MD

The Center for Research and Education, Pediatrix Medical Group,
1301 Concord Terrace, Sunrise, FL 33323, USA

The clinical situation

Anyone who has practiced neonatology for some length of time has encountered the following patient. He (and it usually is a he) starts life as an extremely low birth weight (ELBW) infant with relatively mild lung disease, and typically requires only modest respiratory assistance during the first weeks of life. Along the way, there is a sepsis scare, either in the form of generalized septicemia or necrotizing enterocolitis (NEC), which sets back ventilator weaning for a few days. During this period, feedings are withheld because the infant appears unstable, he often has abdominal distension, and the fragile nature of the baby's illness is all too apparent to both parents and caregivers. After several days of anxious observation, there appears to be a light at the end of the tunnel and the reduction of ventilator support recommences, with everyone's optimism rising as feedings are restarted and weight gain resumes. Often, the infant is extubated to continuous positive airway pressure (CPAP) or oxygen after a period of several days, but the infant's work of breathing appears to be excessive. Efforts by the staff to "cheer-lead" the baby in an attempt to avoid another endotracheal tube inevitably fail, and at some point during a notably bad night, the child is reintubated and mechanical ventilation is started once again. The parents rush to the hospital when they hear the news and are devastated by this turn for the worse, while the physician attempts to reassure them that this is only a temporary setback and the child will soon be extubated again. In most cases, that assessment is accurate, but every once in a while, something else happens, and it is a sequence of events that devastates the family,

E-mail address: alan_spitzer@pediatrix.com

frustrates the medical staff, and seems to last forever. It is "the dreaded desaturating baby syndrome."

The scenario at this point becomes increasingly dark and disturbing. The child is officially diagnosed as having severe bronchopulmonary dysplasia (BPD), according to the most recent criteria [1]. Further attempts to initiate ventilator weaning are not well tolerated, and, in fact, support often begins to increase. At first, it is only a modest increase in oxygen. Then, as the work of breathing progressively increases, with a rise in the respiratory rate and more retractions, the pressures gradually creep upward on the ventilator. The nursing staff begins to complain that they can't do any of the baby's care because he turns blue as soon as you touch him—even changing a diaper provokes a cyanotic episode that occasionally requires hand ventilation for several minutes to allow recovery. Bronchospasm is raised as a possible etiology, but the use of bronchodilators usually fails to improve the clinical situation and increasing numbers of the severe cyanotic spells soon follow. At this point, you realize that this infant will now become a reminder to you for the next several months of the imperfect nature of newborn intensive care and how much we still need to learn about the neonatal patient. This clinical situation forms the focus of discussion for this article.

Etiological considerations

The modern era of neonatal intensive care began in the 1960s, following the death of the infant son of President John Fitzgerald Kennedy in 1963, several months before his assassination. Patrick Bouvier Kennedy was born 5.5 weeks prematurely by caesarean section at the Otis Air Force Base Hospital, with a birth weight of 4 lb, 10.5 oz (2112 g), and was transferred to Massachusetts General Hospital, where he was placed in a hyperbaric oxygen chamber, dying 2 days later of hyaline membrane disease. An obituary in *The New York Times* pointed out that the only treatment available "for a victim of hyaline membrane disease is to monitor the infant's blood chemistry and to try to keep it near normal levels. Thus, the battle for the Kennedy baby was lost only because medical science has not yet advanced far enough to accomplish as quickly as necessary what the body can do by itself in its own time."

Prompted by this tragedy, several physicians around the country (most notably Gluck at Yale, Stahlman at Vanderbilt, and Tooley at UCSF, as well as a few others) began intensive care nurseries that were designed to treat patients such as the Kennedy infant. Initially, the primary focal point of these units was respiratory care, because immature lungs and hyaline membrane disease (now called respiratory distress syndrome, or RDS) were such commonly lethal issues. Inspired by the initial success of Delivoria-Papadopoulos and colleagues [2] in Toronto, who successfully ventilated a neonate with RDS, efforts to improve neonatal ventilatory support began in earnest and quickly emerged as life-saving interventions. At first, survival was the sole concern, but by 1967, a new entity emerged that ultimately became the leading focus of neonatal research during the subsequent 4 decades. That entity, bronchopulmonary dysplasia (BPD), was first characterized by Northway and colleagues [3] in a seminal paper in the *New England Journal of Medicine*, and they attributed the disease primarily to the effects of oxygen on the lung. Subsequent studies of BPD made it clear, however, that oxygen was not the only culprit in this new disease. Intubation and positive pressure ventilation, when used for a period of time, also seemed intrinsically related to the development of BPD [4,5].

As increasing numbers of infants with BPD survived, the management of these patients became a major concern in newborn medicine. Attempts to aggressively and quickly reduce ventilator support in the chronically ventilated patient often resulted either in death or cor pulmonale [6]. The ongoing use, however, of oxygen and positive pressure ventilation seemed inherently wrong, because these factors, while necessary to keep the infant alive, were the same agents that appeared to cause the disease itself. More importantly, neonatologists began to recognize and attempt to cope with the debilitating effects of BPD on the neonate and the family: pulmonary fibrosis, electrolyte and acid-base disturbances, nutritional and growth failure, osteopenia, increased infections, developmental delay, cerebral palsy, social interactive problems, and numerous other long-term consequences emerged as issues with which the neonatologist and the pediatrician were forced to contend [7–9].

In addition to the previously mentioned complications, a significant number of these infants frequently had episodes that alarmed everyone. These events, referred to as "BPD spells," could strike fear into even the most seasoned neonatal nurse. In their most acute form, an infant could die within minutes. The child would appear to be stable and resting comfortably on the ventilator, but within minutes, often unprovoked, the infant would become rapidly and progressively cyanotic. Hand ventilation would often appear not to move any air into the chest at all and breath sounds would be absent. Fearing that the endotracheal (ET) tube was plugged, the neonatologist would rapidly change the tube, only to find that it was completely clear and that ongoing ventilation, even at extraordinarily high pressures, would barely move the chest. At this stage, one of two things might happen: the child might die, or he would very slowly return back to baseline, completely terrifying everyone who witnessed the episode. In other cases, the deterioration was less acute, but the ability to get back to baseline was often as difficult as that seen in the acutely deteriorating patient. While in the modern era, the type of infant who develops BPD has changed, with the ELBW infant now forming the primary BPD population, the presence of desaturation episodes remains an ongoing issue in neonatology. The questions, therefore, about these desaturations persist: what exactly is occurring, what triggers these spells, how should they be treated, and, most importantly, is there any way they can be avoided?

Pathophysiology of the acutely desaturation infant

Two diagnostic approaches to these desaturation spells, which unfortunately are not used very often in current practice, provide some answers to the pathophysiology of the acute cyanotic episode in the infant with BPD: neonatal pulmonary function testing (PFT) and bedside flexible fiber-optic bronchoscopy. Before the introduction of computerized technology, the performance of PFTs was difficult and complicated. As computerized bedside technology progressed, studies to define the pathophysiological changes in many clinical circumstances were initiated to better understand the clinically observed abnormalities. Later, the introduction of computerized graphics monitoring as a component of modern ventilators essentially replaced stand-alone PFT devices. Although they are not quite as sophisticated, ventilator graphics do provide a wealth of information that is invaluable in assessing and understanding the respiratory condition of the neonate.

Computerized PFT testing in a neonate is somewhat different from PFT testing in an adult. Because of the inability of the neonate to cooperate with the procedure, some alterations in the basic approach must be performed. In trying to understand neonatal lung mechanics, the primary components that one is typically interested in are compliance (stiffness) of the lung, resistance in the airways, and flow-volume relationships during breathing. These measurements can be made through the use of the following tools: a pressure transducer that measures flow in and out of the lungs during a defined period of time; an esophageal balloon that provides a reasonable valuation of transthoracic pressure with respiration; and a computer to record and analyze the respiratory cycle (Figs. 1 and 2).

In the study of these infants who had frequent decreases in oxygen saturation, several characteristics could be discerned. First, dynamic lung compliance (the change in volume divided by the change in pressure during a respiratory cycle) is typically reduced, indicative of a lung that has been

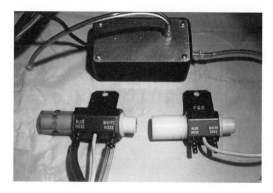

Fig. 1. Illustration of pressure transducer (top) and neonatal and pediatric pneumotachographs (bottom) used in the performance of pulmonary function testing in infants.

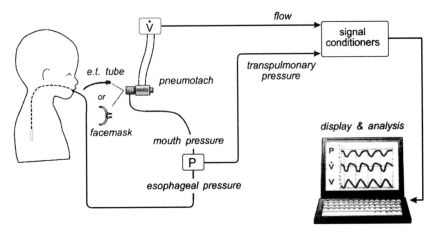

Fig. 2. Set-up for performing neonatal pulmonary function tests. The infant breathes through a face mask or the ET tube into a pneumotachograph, which senses the change in flow and converts it to an electrical signal, which can be recorded on the computer. The esophageal balloon, placed approximately 3 to 5 cm above the lower esophageal sphincter, provides an approximation of intrathoracic pressure change through the pressure transducer, also noted on the computer graphics. One then has a measure of flow per unit time and simultaneous pressure change, from which dynamic pulmonary function measurements can be performed. (*Courtesy of* V. K. Bhutani, MD, Palo Alto, California.)

injured through the use of mechanical ventilation for a significant period of time (Fig. 3). When compliance is decreased, it subsequently requires additional effort to inflate the lung, often precipitating further elevation of ventilator settings. Airway resistance (the change in pressure divided by the change in flow) is also consistently elevated in this patient population (Fig. 4).

Of interest in this respect, however, is that while lung compliance in neonates with pulmonary disease is commonly reduced, the compliance of the airway is often increased. Neonatal airways were never designed to see the positive pressures that are often required to inflate an atelectatic lung with RDS. The consequence of mechanical ventilation is that in the process of

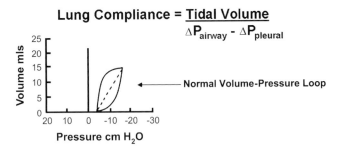

Fig. 3. Pulmonary compliance calculation from neonatal pulmonary function testing.

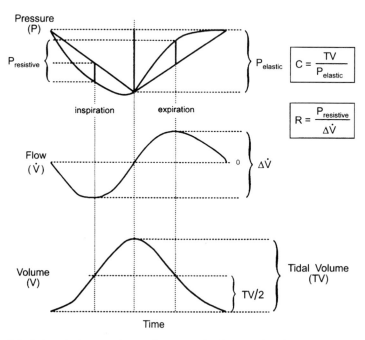

Fig. 4. Calculation of airway resistance in neonatal pulmonary functions. A single breath is shown in the figure, with the methods for calculating both compliance and resistance. It should be noted that compliance is calculated at the point of zero flow, whereas resistance is measured at the point of maximum flow during either inspiration or expiration, which may differ significantly. A linear respiratory model is assumed. (*From* Abassi S, Sivieri EM, Bhutani VK. Evaluation of pulmonary function in a neonate. In: Polin RA, Fox WW, Abman SH, editors. Fetal and neonatal physiology. 3rd edition. Philadelphia: W. B. Saunders Co, Inc; 2004. p. 923; with permission.)

reaching an opening pressure for the lung, the larger airways are overdistended with each ventilatory cycle, resulting in increased airway compliance as the tracheal cartilaginous rings are insufficiently developed to cope with these pressures. One must also remember that normal breathing is produced by the creation of a negative pressure within the airway, not through the delivery of a positive pressure breath to the airways and lungs. Because the pulmonary component of compliance is so much more significant in neonatal pulmonary function measurements than the airway component, however, the airway contribution to compliance is often masked and unappreciated until frequent desaturations begin to occur. Similarly, early in the course of neonatal lung disease, resistance alterations are modest and underappreciated, since the airways are stented open by the pressure delivered during ventilatory assistance. As pressures are reduced over time, however, the resistance, particularly expiratory resistance, increases and becomes a major contributor to the clinical problem of desaturation described earlier. The key issue that must be resolved is a determination of how much of the airway problem is a result of increased airway reactivity, and how much is the result of increased compliance from overstretching during prolonged ventilatory support and tracheobronchomalacia.

With the use of pulmonary function testing, a series of steps can be taken to determine the cause of the desaturations that are being observed. Baseline compliance and resistance measurements can be made, and the flow-volume loop in the infant can be examined. Depending on the gestational age and the current age of the infant, normal levels of compliance and resistance have been reported [10]. Flow-volume loops in infants with BPD have characteristic appearances that can provide clues to the etiology of the desaturation episodes (Fig. 5). Whether an infant is spontaneously breathing or remains on ventilatory assistance, these loops provide indication of both elevated pressures and/or complete airway collapse, particularly during the expiratory cycle of breathing. As seen in Fig. 6, the patient with BPD will often show a dramatic slowing of airflow during expiration, and, if tracheobronchomalacia is present, zero flow will often be seen. This type of acute, complete obstruction, in my experience, is the predominant pattern seen in the infant with frequent desaturation episodes and characteristic of the significant airway injury that may be present.

The mechanism that triggers these events is not as easily assessed, but can again be discerned from PFTs and bronchoscopy. Whereas the focus in BPD is typically on the lung and lung growth, the degree of airway injury remains an important factor. In addition to the stretching and increase in airway compliance that results in a loss of overall tone, cilia in the larger airway are injured and excessive mucous production is observed in response to the presence of an ET tube and positive pressure ventilation (PPV). This mucous tends to be very thick and tenacious, is often difficult to remove even with vigorous suctioning, and frequently occludes the mainstem bronchi and bronchioles. In the airway with malacia and thick mucous, further loss of tone within the airway (which may be acute with agitation and crying, or slowly progressive during sleep) prevents the airway of the infant from reopening as the thick mucous causes the walls of the airway to adhere. On numerous occasions, under direct visualization with bronchoscopy, we have observed airway collapse and wall adherence, which could not be reopened with PPV. Only the insertion of either the bronchoscope itself or a suction catheter through the mucous allowed the airway to re-expand. It appears that this physiology is present during many instances of acute desaturation in infants with BPD.

Confirmation of this pathophysiology is observed during bronchoscopy, as indicated. Flexible fiber-optic bronchoscopy is an ideal tool for revealing the dynamics of lung pathophysiology in these circumstances. This bronchoscopy can be performed at the bedside under appropriate sedation, and does not require a trip to the operating room. Bronchoscopy can be performed with a 2.2- or 2.5-mm scope, which readily enters a 3.0 endotracheal tube. The bronchoscope allows video recording, which is extremely helpful in reviewing the findings with the medical staff and parents at a later time. In

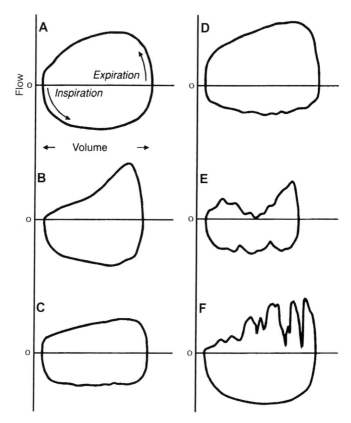

Fig. 5. Changes in appearance of flow-volume loops during neonatal pulmonary function testing. (*A*) Normal flow-volume loop. (*B*) Infant with increased expiratory resistance, usually from extrathoracic upper airway obstruction. (*C*) Infant with fixed upper airway obstruction. (*D*) Inspiratory limitation seen with small airway disease or with tracheal granuloma. (*E*) Tracheobronchomalacia. (*F*) Increased airway secretions or water in the ventilator tubing. (*From* Abassi S, Sivieri EM, Bhutani VK. Evaluation of pulmonary function in a neonate. In: Polin RA, Fox WW, Abman SH, editors. Fetal and neonatal physiology. 3rd edition. Philadelphia: W. B. Saunders Co, Inc; 2004. p. 924; with permission.)

a normal airway below the glottic opening, there is a characteristic appearance, as seen in Fig. 7: the cartilaginous rings are readily observed, there is no airway edema or mucous, the carina is sharply defined, and the mainstem bronchi are oval in shape.

In virtually every intubated premature infant, however, within a few days of intubation and initiation of pulmonary toilet, several changes begin to appear that are consistent: the carina thickens and becomes much broader in configuration, a granuloma begins to form, usually at the take-off of the right mainstem bronchus, mucous production increases, and the bronchi themselves become flattened and more elongated in shape (Fig. 8). The airway is often patent for a lesser portion of the day under these conditions.

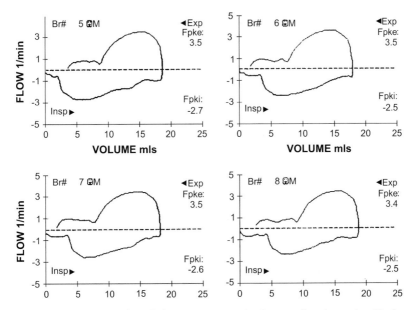

Fig. 6. Severe tracheobronchomalacia seen on neonatal pulmonary function testing. During expiration, there is repeated obstruction of flow during expiration (above the dotted line). Limitation of inspiratory flow is also seen (below the dotted line), as a result of a large tracheal granuloma.

The granuloma appears to arise from a combination of ET suctioning and infant movement that repeatedly repositions the ET tube within the airway, irritating the carina. Since the right mainstem bronchus lies in a straighter line to the direction of the trachea, the ET tube, and the suction catheter, it is the area just to the right of the mainstem bronchus that typically suffers the brunt of the airway trauma during airway management and pulmonary toilet. The granulomas that form can occasionally be quite large in size, in some cases completely occluding a bronchus. These granulomas are remarkably responsive to corticosteroid therapy, and we have seen them shrink and nearly disappear within days of initiating treatment for an occluded airway. The PFT pattern in such cases reveals very low flow during inspiration.

As the duration of intubation and PPV progress, the mainstem bronchi continue to flatten, at times appearing slit-like in their configuration, as the tone of the airway decreases and mucous production increases. During bronchoscopy, although the child is sedated, stimulation of the airway will occasionally result in observable collapse to the point that the airway becomes a pinhole through which air entry is negligible. In such circumstances, it is little wonder that acute cyanosis occurs. Furthermore, when the child becomes hypoxemic, agitation often increases. Crying, which is a phenomenon of expiration only, forces the airway closed even further, and a vicious cycle is initiated that is difficult to interrupt. Last, there is evidence in some

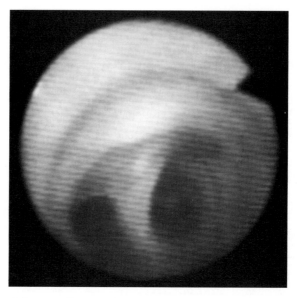

Fig. 7. A normal airway on fiber-optic bronchoscopy. The carina is narrow and the mainstem bronchi are well-shaped ovals. The tracheal rings can be seen, there is no hemorrhage in the airway, and there is little evidence of mucous. (Note: the faint horizontal lines are a moiré pattern from the video screen.)

infants that with this type of airway collapse, pulmonary arterial pressure increases in the face of hypoxemia, and the combination of loss of airway tone and increased pulmonary vascular resistance is a particularly difficult situation for both infant and physician (Fig. 9). Tracheobronchomalacia, therefore, is an especially serious issue for the chronically ventilated patient, and a relatively common circumstance in the infant who has severe ongoing desaturation problems.

Although tracheobronchomalacia is the event of greatest concern, increased airway reactivity does affect some infants and may be helped by bronchodilators. The flow-volume pattern in these infants is different, however, and the progressive response to bronchodilators can be charted from observation of both the flow-volume loop and the decrease in airway resistance that can be seen in response to the bronchodilating agent.

In each of the above clinical situations, one must also be aware that certain "triggering" events may be present that will also need evaluation and treatment. Septicemia may initially manifest by altering airway tone and result in more frequent desaturation. Biochemical disturbances such as hypoglycemia, hypocalcemia, hypokalemia, and so forth, may also initiate events that result in hypoxemia, either through airway alteration, or separately by themselves through hypoventilation and decreased gas exchange as the infant becomes stressed. Although one might anticipate that obstructive apnea may present with recurring hypoxemia, it is more common in our experience

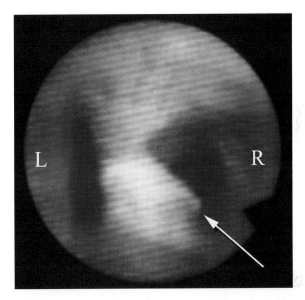

Fig. 8. Initial changes observed in ventilated patients on flexible fiber-optic bronchoscopy. A granuloma has formed at the take-off to the right main stem bronchus, indicated by an arrow. The bronchi are more oval in shape than normal, the carina is thickened in appearance, and the airways are slightly hyperemic.

for the apnea associated with severe airway obstruction to appear central in origin, with the infant ceasing to breathe. Careful evaluation of the patient is always indicated in the face of frequent severe hypoxemic spells.

Approach to evaluation of the child with severe, recurring hypoxemia

In any infant with recurring episodes on oxygen desaturation and cyanosis, the following steps should be performed. First, one must determine if it is the infant or a mechanical problem that is provoking these events, and restore the infant's oxygenation as quickly as possible. The infant should be disconnected from the ventilator and hand ventilated while the ventilator circuit is checked for any possible malfunctions. Occasionally, one may find that the desired ventilator pressures are simply not being met and there is a leak in the ventilator circuit. Exposure of the infant to such variability may precipitate periods of agitation and desaturation until a more stable ventilator environment can be provided.

Once the ventilator is determined to be performing as expected, attention should be given to the possible causes on neonatal problems. It is not easy to provide a list of etiologies here, since almost any clinical or metabolic abnormality in a chronically ventilated neonate may produce episodes of desaturation if timely intervention does not occur. Some of the more common

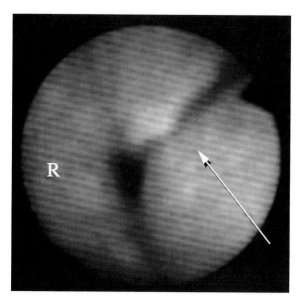

Fig. 9. Severe tracheobronchomalacia in a 3-month-old infant. The trachea folds upon itself into a buckled position, narrowing the lumen of the mainstem bronchi in the process to a fraction of normal size. The arrow points to the folded trachea.

nonpulmonary causes, however, deserve mention. Sepsis and pneumonia, the most immediately treatable etiologies, should always be considered first if an infant presents with a sudden change in frequency of acute cyanotic episodes. Blood cultures, a complete blood count (CBC) with differential and platelet count, and a C-reactive protein may all be helpful in defining the presence or absence of bacterial sepsis. Examination of tracheal aspirates for culture and white blood cells may also be helpful in diagnosing pneumonia or tracheitis, both of which can provoke more frequent desaturations. Tracheitis may arise from chronic use of the endotracheal tube, and is usually an inflammatory response to either irritation or infection, marked by elevated white blood cells in the tracheal aspirate. With a tracheitis, the secretions often increase dramatically and interfere with ventilation and oxygenation, yet the initial chest radiographs may not reveal any significant change.

It has also been our observation over many years, however, that one of the more likely causes of a sepsis-like syndrome in a neonate, although often not easily diagnosed, is viral infection. Especially during the winter months in the colder climates, one can usually assume that 10% or more of the nursery care providers are infected with a viral respiratory infection (in the summer, viral gastrointestinal infections can act similarly). It is simply not possible to exclude all of these individuals from delivering care, and, in many instances, personnel are clinically asymptomatic, even though they may be shedding virus at the time. In the neonate, the clinical response to a viral infection may be indistinguishable from a bacterial event, with the production of circulating cytokines and other vasoactive mediators, all of which produce the clinical signs of a sepsis-like picture. In most instances, the bouts of cyanosis are more limited than those seen with bacterial infection, but the underlying clinical condition of the infant can nonetheless be adversely affected for some time by a viral infection.

Metabolic abnormalities, such as hypoglycemia, hypokalemia, hypo- or hypercalcemia, hypo- or hypermagnesemia, and acid-base disturbances can all result in increased problems with saturation and cyanosis. In the chronically ventilated BPD patient, one of the more common clinical situations that can develop is that of respiratory acidosis and compensatory metabolic alkalosis. With careful attention to the monitoring of electrolytes, these abnormalities are not usually difficult to manage. The introduction of diuretic therapy, however, can aggravate the situation by worsening the alkalosis. In an effort to adjust the pH to a more normal range, the infant may additionally compensate by further slowing respiration. Apnea and cyanosis may then increase, even though the problem is metabolic in origin. Correction of this degree of severe acid-base abnormality is not easy, and one should consider the necessity of using diuretics, especially on a daily basis. Also, we have observed that the thiazide diuretics, commonly used in conjunction with spironolactone, may be more likely to worsen alkalosis in neonates than is seen with intermittent use of furosemide. Regardless of the diuretic choice, early initiation of potassium chloride supplementation may help avoid this problem. It is not uncommon for caregivers to overlook KCl supplementation until the acid-base problem is evident, and one should start KCl early rather than later, once diuretics are begun.

When the circuit, infectious causes, and metabolic and acid-base issues have been eliminated, one should focus on the lung and airway. The first step in assessing the situation is to review the frequency and severity of episodes of desaturation, especially with the bedside nursing staff. Their description will often be helpful in sorting out the problem. At times, the desaturations are not as severe as they initially seem and the infant's agitation may actually reflect clinical improvement and a demonstration on the part of the infant to have the ET tube removed, suggesting that one can consider extubation to CPAP.

More commonly, however, increasing desaturations are evidence of some form of respiratory deterioration. A chest radiograph is essential in evaluating whether there has been a significant lung problem that needs to be addressed. In the infant with BPD, shifting atelectasis and hyperinflation may be responsible for the clinical hypoxemia. Alternatively, the infant may have a pneumonia that acts in a similar fashion. Sudden loss of lung volume may lead to acute deterioration in blood gases with desaturation and hypercarbia. It should not be forgotten, however, that while the lung demonstrates atelectasis on x ray, it may actually be an alteration in the airway that initiates the change.

To assess the airway, one should examine either neonatal pulmonary functions or pulmonary graphics on the ventilator's respiratory monitor, both of which reveal much critical information in this regard. One should see if compliance is reduced and whether resistance has increased. Resistance, in particular, must be carefully evaluated. Flow-volume loops should be studied to see if only expiratory resistance is increased, or whether inspiratory resistance is also affected. An increase in inspiratory resistance usually reflects an anatomical lesion, such as a granuloma, that limits air entry into the lung. Increased expiratory resistance is usually attributable to one of two diagnoses: tracheobronchomalacia or increased airway reactivity with bronchospasm. In tracheobronchomalacia, air flow on flow-volume loops will notably be seen to acutely drop to zero flow during the expiratory cycle. With increased airway reactivity, flow drops rapidly and expiration may be prolonged, but usually does not go to zero flow.

Occasionally, it is not possible to distinguish bronchomalacia from bronchospasm on pulmonary graphics or pulmonary functions alone. In such cases, flexible fiber-optic bronchoscopy should be used to make the diagnosis. Although bronchospasm is not easy to see on bronchoscopy, airway injury and collapse of the airway with tracheobronchomalacia is usually readily observed, as are any granulomas that might be limiting inspiratory flow (granulomas do not often obstruct during expiration). In addition, once the diagnosis of tracheobronchomalacia is made with PFT testing, the response to care can be judged by gradually increasing end expiratory pressure to view normalization of the flow-volume loop. During bronchoscopy, the same response can be directly observed by seeing what level of end expiratory pressure maintains airway caliber. The airway can be seen to enlarge dramatically to a normal caliber once the critical opening pressure for the compliant airway is achieved.

Management of the infant with frequent desaturation

As is true in all of medicine, appropriate management cannot be initiated until the correct diagnosis is made. Because of the unstable nature of the infant with ongoing desaturation, diagnostic studies are often deferred until the patient is more "stable." This approach is usually unsuccessful and one must then initiate a diagnostic evaluation at a time when the infant is actually less stable than was true at an earlier point in the course of care. Frequent desaturations are abnormal and must be evaluated as soon as they are clinically a concern. The long-term effects of recurring hypoxemia on neurodevelopment, even when brief, can be significant.

As with many neonatal problems, the initial diagnostic approach to recurring frequent desaturations is somewhat nonspecific. Typical studies should include the following:

- Chest and abdominal radiograph
- CBC with differential and platelet count

- Blood culture
- Serum electrolytes
- Calcium, magnesium, phosphate
- Arterial blood gases
    - Pulse oximetry and end-tidal CO_2 monitoring may be helpful
- C-reactive protein (if sepsis is suspected)
- Apnea assessment
- Pulmonary function tests or pulmonary graphics monitor evaluation
    - Pre- and postbronchodilator
- Bronchoscopy, as indicated

More specific biochemical evaluation for sepsis and other inflammatory processes through tandem mass spectroscopy evaluation for sepsis may be of value in the not-too-distant future. Correction of biochemical abnormalities, especially those seen in acid-base disturbances, may significantly aid in reducing periods of desaturation. As noted previously, the most common situation that produces problems is seen in the child with severe respiratory acidosis and compensatory metabolic alkalosis who then is treated with diuretics. As the child hypoventilates further to reduce the pH, hypoxemia may occur with greater frequency.

If one has eliminated the possible biochemical and infectious causes of desaturation, management of the child's airway emerges as a critical and somewhat controversial issue. If bronchospasm is present, although not common, treatment with bronchodilator therapy is appropriate. One must be cautious, however, in that neonates, as is true of older children and adults, do become tachyphylactic to doses of these agents, and increasing frequency of treatment and higher doses may become necessary. When this evolution of the process occurs, however, reevaluation of the etiology may be indicated, as the bronchospasm may have actually been a manifestation of early tracheobronchomalacia, which is now more clinically evident.

For the infant with tracheobronchomalacia, several steps can be helpful. Most importantly, the recovery from this problem is not quick, and the physician should make the family aware that it is likely to be weeks or months before sufficient cartilage and growth have been added to the airway to maintain adequate patency, especially with crying. Since growth is a critical contributing factor, nutritional considerations are of paramount importance. In the modern era, in which both alveolar growth and somatic growth in neonates with BPD appear to be inhibited, the focus on nutrition cannot be overemphasized. High-caloric density formula can be of great help in assisting recovery, and nutritional consultation may be of great benefit to the infant. The recent introduction of 30-calorie Special Care formula by Ross Laboratories may be of great value in improving calories for growth and not just for breathing.

With respect to pulmonary care, if the infant has been ventilated with a pressure-controlled ventilator, switching to a volume ventilator, or, on some devices, switching to a volume-delivery mode may be all that is necessary. In many chronically ventilated patients, as they gain in strength, inconsistency of volume delivery to the lung with each breath may provoke episodes of agitation and crying, which will rapidly worsen the ensuing hypoxemia. A consistent volume delivery or guaranteed volume ventilation may overcome this issue. The clinician, however, needs to be aware that, occasionally, periods of high pressure are needed to deliver those volumes, and the pressure should not be limited to any significant degree. As the infant recovers, and the trachea matures, weaning can occur.

Another approach that may be helpful in some infants with tracheobronchomalacia is progressively elevating the positive end expiratory pressure (PEEP) to reduce the potential for airway collapse. In some situations, a PEEP of 12 to 15 cm H_2O may be needed to stabilize the airway, but even then, a child may Valsalva and overcome this end-expiratory pressure. In general, however, higher PEEP does permit a greater period of the day to be spent at a more tolerable level of oxygenation. It is unclear if the provision of such an extraordinary PEEP in a young infant further damages the injured airway, but some infants will become far easier for the nurses to care for with this approach. Again, with appropriate nutritional support, growth will eventually allow recovery in most cases. Furthermore, some exciting new approaches are currently being examined that may alter the recovery process as well. The administration of growth factors may soon enhance the recovery from this situation and significantly shorten the length of hospital stay [11].

We have also found it helpful to have a consistent group of caregivers for infants with severe airway instability. The nursing staff get to know and understand the patient well, work with the family to assist them through a very difficult period in the neonatal intensive care unit that may last months, and provide optimal feedback to the physician about the infant so that weaning can eventually occur. The dedication of a specific care team can be very helpful in managing care for both the infant and the family in this highly charged clinical situation.

Summary

The infant with frequent desaturations may have a variety of causes for these events. Frequent hypoxemia should always be viewed as a significant change in the clinical status of the patient and must be investigated carefully for possible etiology. When many of the common extra-airway causes for desaturation are ruled out, one should attempt to distinguish between central apnea and obstructive events. The most commonly overlooked obstructive event is tracheobronchomalacia, and steps should be initiated to understand the scope of the problem through pulmonary function testing and bronchoscopy. One should also provide adequate respiratory support for the infant until adequate time passes to enable airway growth and improved cartilaginous deposition to occur. Parents must be carefully supported during this difficult time, because the stress of having an infant who requires prolonged hospitalization and care for tracheobronchomalacia is substantial.

References

[1] Walsh MC, Yao Q, Gettner P, et al, for National Institute of Child Health and Human Development Neonatal Research Network. Impact of a physiologic definition on bronchopulmonary dysplasia rates. Pediatrics 2004;114(5):1305–11.

[2] Delivoria-Papadopoulos M, Levison H, Swyer PR. Intermittent positive pressure respiration as a treatment in severe respiratory distress syndrome. Arch Dis Child 1965;40:474–9.

[3] Northway WH Jr, Rosan RC, Porter DY. Pulmonary disease following respirator therapy of hyaline-membrane disease. Bronchopulmonary dysplasia. N Engl J Med 1967;276:357–68.

[4] Philip AG. Oxygen plus pressure plus time: the etiology of bronchopulmonary dysplasia. Pediatrics 1975;55:44–50.

[5] Berg TJ, Pagtakhan RD, Reed MH, et al. Bronchopulmonary dysplasia and lung rupture in hyaline membrane disease: influence of continuous distending pressure. Pediatrics 1975;55: 51–4.

[6] Hislop AA, Haworth SG. Related articles, pulmonary vascular damage and the development of cor pulmonale following hyaline membrane disease. Pediatr Pulmonol 1990;9:152–61.

[7] Moon NM, Mohay HA, Gray PH. Developmental patterns from 1 to 4 years of extremely preterm infants who required home oxygen therapy. Early Hum Dev 2006; [epub Jul 21].

[8] Bhandari A, Panitch HB. Pulmonary outcomes in bronchopulmonary dysplasia. Semin Perinatol 2006;30(4):219–26.

[9] Bott L, Beghin L, Devos P, et al. Nutritional status at 2 years in former infants with bronchopulmonary dysplasia influences nutrition and pulmonary outcomes during childhood. Pediatr Res 2006;60:340–4.

[10] Siveri EM, Bhutani VK. Pulmonary mechanics. In: Donn SM, Sinha SK, editors. Neonatal respiratory care. Philadelphia: Elsevier Mosby; 2006. p. 57–8.

[11] Asikainen TM, Chang LY, Coalson JJ, et al. Improved lung growth and function through hypoxia-inducible factor in primate chronic lung disease of prematurity. FASEB J 2006; 20:1698–700.

ELSEVIER
SAUNDERS

CLINICS IN
PERINATOLOGY

Clin Perinatol 34 (2007) 73–92

Continuous Positive Airway Pressure and Noninvasive Ventilation

Sherry E. Courtney, MD, MS[a],*,
Keith J. Barrington, MD[b]

[a]Division of Neonatology, Schneider Children's Hospital, North Shore Long Island Jewish Health System, Room 344, 269-01 76th Avenue, New Hyde Park, New York 11040, USA
[b]Division of Neonatology, Neonatal Intensive Care Unit, McGill University, Royal Victoria Hospital, 687 Pine Avenue, Montreal, Quebec H3A1A1, Canada

Noninvasive ventilation

What is the best way to treat an infant requiring ventilatory support? How can we minimize damage to the lungs and airways while treating the underlying disorder? We do not yet have all the answers to these important questions. Respiratory support without endotracheal intubation is an attractive option. In this article the authors review the different methods of providing continuous positive airway pressure (CPAP) and more complex forms of noninvasive ventilation (NIV), such as bilevel CPAP and nasal intermittent mandatory ventilation (NIMV).

Back to the future

In the 1960s and early 1970s intubation and ventilation of infants, especially premature infants, was largely experimental. The authors recall the death of President Kennedy's son Patrick, born at 34 weeks' gestation in 1963 at a weight of more than 2 kg, from respiratory distress syndrome (RDS). More than 40 years later, death of such an infant is nearly inconceivable. Early attempts at ventilation were cumbersome, hampered by lack of appropriate equipment, and could be likened to hanging a picture using a forklift. One author (SEC) recalls that, while she was a medical student, an intermittent positive pressure ventilation device used to give inhalation treatments to adults provided positive pressure to intubated newborns,

* Corresponding author.
E-mail address: scourtne@lij.edu (S.E. Courtney).

0095-5108/07/$ - see front matter © 2007 Elsevier Inc. All rights reserved.
doi:10.1016/j.clp.2006.12.008 *perinatology.theclinics.com*

and end-expiratory pressure was given by submersing the expiratory tubing into a cylinder taped to the wall and filled with water.

When infant ventilators became commonplace, the water cylinders disappeared. No one could have foreseen these precursors of bubble CPAP reincarnated in the last years of the twentieth century. The bubble CPAP device described by Gregory and colleagues [1] in their classic 1971 article was fashioned not from any belief that bubble CPAP was particularly good, but from the fact no other way to provide CPAP to newborns was easily available at that time.

In fact, it is not CPAP and NIV that are new, but our interest in them. It is true that at first we had no good way to provide CPAP if infants were not intubated. Face masks were sometimes used, strapped in place around the infant's head. The pressure required to obtain a good seal was considerable, and severe molding of the head ensued. In the days before availability of cranial sonography, the effect these masks had on the incidence of intracranial hemorrhage was unknown, but we suspect the effect was not beneficial. Use of nasal prongs to provide CPAP was described by Kattwinkel and colleagues [2] in 1973, shortly after Gregory's article was published. As infant ventilators appeared on the scene and began multiplying in number and design, neonatologists became fascinated with the new "toys." Many neglected CPAP altogether, and indeed, in the pre-surfactant and pre-antenatal steroid era, infant ventilators saved many lives.

We knew little, however, about how best to manage infants on ventilators. As with many situations in which randomized controlled trials are difficult, long, and expensive, strategies of management grew out of experience and opinion. A multitude of magic numbers appeared: intubate all babies of X weight, do not extubate until Y weight, do not use end-expiratory pressure greater than Z, and so forth. The appearance of high-frequency ventilation in the 1980s added another level of complexity to infant ventilation, and more machines to our armamentarium. NICUs built more than 15 or 20 years ago can often barely accommodate the equipment needed at many bedsides today.

The era of invasive mechanical ventilation as the best and only answer to the infant who has respiratory problems came to an end as knowledge increased and technology improved. Data on the fragility of the lung, the cascade of deleterious effects resulting from volutrauma, barotrauma, atelectrauma, and biotrauma coincided to a large extent with more sophisticated infant ventilators that allowed us to synchronize breaths and measure tidal volume. At the same time, interest was renewed in ways that might minimize lung damage by never introducing an endotracheal tube in the first place: NIV.

Continuous positive airway pressure

CPAP is used predominantly for maintaining lung expansion in conditions in which the alveoli tend to collapse or fill with fluid. These conditions include RDS, postextubation and postoperative respiratory management, meconium and other aspiration syndromes, transient tachypnea of the newborn, pulmonary edema, congestive heart failure, pneumonia, resuscitation in the delivery room, high chest wall compliance (such as with extreme prematurity), and pulmonary hemorrhage. CPAP is also used to treat apnea of prematurity, whereby it may stimulate breathing or help maintain airway patency [3]. In laryngomalacia, tracheomalacia, or bronchomalacia CPAP may help stent the airways open, allowing management of the airway without intubation.

Despite the many years since CPAP use was first described in neonates, little is known about how best to use it. We are still uncertain as to whether it should be applied immediately in the delivery room, whether it should be used before or after surfactant administration, and at what levels of positive pressure it should be used. Another uncertainty is whether CPAP or positive end-expiratory pressure (PEEP) is best and under what circumstances. Further confusion is added by the fact that not all CPAP devices are created equal. A multitude of ways to deliver CPAP now exists, and few studies have looked at physiologic or clinical effects of the various devices.

Continuous positive airway pressure apparatus

In general, CPAP can be provided by devices that vary the CPAP level predominantly by a mechanism other than flow variation (continuous flow devices) or by devices that vary CPAP level predominantly by varying the flow rate (variable flow devices).

Continuous flow continuous positive airway pressure

Continuous flow devices use a constant flow and vary the CPAP level by some other mechanism. Infant ventilators are commonly used for continuous flow CPAP. CPAP is increased or decreased, in general, by varying the ventilator's expiratory orifice size. The exhalation valve works in conjunction with other controls, such as flow control and pressure transducers, to maintain the CPAP at the desired level. Bubble CPAP is another form of continuous flow CPAP; the level of pressure is changed by submerging the expiratory limb of the tubing into a water chamber to the depth of the desired CPAP (Fig. 1). Flow, however, may need to be increased if the CPAP level is increased to assure a continuous bubbling in the water chamber, and increasing the flow rate increases the CPAP generated at the nasal prongs, as described below.

Variable flow continuous positive airway pressure

Variable flow CPAP uses flow changes to generate the CPAP level. Special prongs and flow generators are used for variable flow CPAP. One CPAP device that is popular in Scandinavia uses variable flow to generate variable CPAP pressure, which can be delivered by single or binasal prongs, a mask, or an endotracheal tube [4]. Relatively high gas flows are needed.

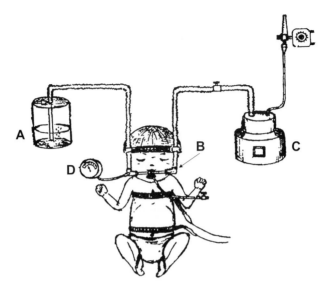

Fig. 1. Schematic of bubble NCPAP delivery system. (*A*) Underwater bubble chamber. (*B*) Nasal CPAP prongs. (*C*) Heated humidifier attached to oxygen blender and flowmeter. (*D*) Manometer. (*Modified from* Liptsen E, Aghai ZH, Pyon KH, et al. Work of breathing during nasal continuous positive airway pressure in preterm infants: a comparison of bubble vs variable flow. J Perinatol 2005;25:453–8; with permission.)

Another popular variable flow device uses a flow driver and special CPAP nosepiece and prongs. The twin jet injector nozzles help maintain a stable mean airway pressure, the prong design allows infant exhalation to redirect the gas flow out the expiratory limb rather than toward the infant, and CPAP pressure is changed by varying the flow to the driver (Fig. 2) [5,6].

Continuous positive airway pressure prongs

Prongs used for CPAP delivery vary considerably. Single nasal prongs, binasal prongs, long nasal prongs, and an endotracheal tube situated in the pharynx have all been used and new prong designs are constantly being produced. Few data exist comparing prong designs; what is available suggests that binasal prongs may be preferable to single nasal prongs [7]. Some CPAP devices, such as the flow drivers, require special prongs used only with the particular flow driver system; other devices, such as bubble CPAP and ventilator-generated continuous flow CPAP, can use various commercially available CPAP prongs.

Comparative studies

Continuous positive airway pressure versus other interventions

Few randomized trials evaluating CPAP in neonates have been done. Cochrane reviews on prophylactic CPAP and CPAP for resuscitation found

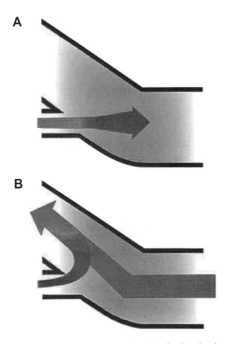

Fig. 2. Design of nosepiece for variable flow NCPAP. (*A*) On inspiration gas is entrained help-ing to create a stable mean airway pressure. (*B*) On expiration the prong design redirects gas flow out the expiratory limb rather than toward the infant. (*Courtesy of* Viasys Healthcare, Inc., Conshohocken, PA; with permission.)

insufficient evidence for any conclusions [8,9]. Additionally, given the wide use of antenatal steroids and exogenous surfactant after 1990, studies done before that date may not be totally relevant to today's population of preterm infants. Cochrane reviews on CPAP for RDS and early versus de-layed use of CPAP for RDS point this out as a major difficulty [10,11]. Nonetheless, some of these trials are of interest given today's controversy regarding when to use surfactant if CPAP is applied early. In a 1976 report, Krouskop and colleagues [12] found no difference in survival or complica-tions in infants assigned randomly to early (fraction of inspired oxygen [F_{IO_2}] requirement 0.40) or late CPAP (F_{IO_2} requirement 0.70); however, these infants were large by today's standards (mean birth weight > 1700 g). Simi-larly, Han and coworkers [13] found no differences in outcome in 82 infants less than 32 weeks' gestation who were randomly assigned to CPAP at birth or CPAP when F_{IO_2} reached greater than 0.50. These infants were somewhat smaller than those reported by Krouskop (mean approximately 1300 g). One is tempted to cautiously conclude from these older studies that in the absence of surfactant therapy, CPAP alone may not be of great benefit.

Some support for this conclusion is lent by the post–surfactant-era trial by Verder and colleagues [14]. Sixty-eight infants were randomly assigned to receive surfactant then CPAP, or CPAP alone. Median birth weight was approximately 1300 g. Although the study was relatively small and included many large preterm infants, those infants treated with surfactant then CPAP did better (less requirement for subsequent mechanical ventilation) than those treated with CPAP alone. Recently, however, Sandri and colleagues [15] randomly assigned 230 infants 28 to 31 weeks' gestation to prophylactic (within 30 minutes of birth) or rescue ($FiO_2 > 0.40$) nasal CPAP. There was no difference between groups in surfactant therapy, need for mechanical ventilation, or air leaks. Larger trials addressing the issue of when surfactant is indicated in the infant managed with CPAP are now in progress.

There are several other trials that used less rigorous designs, such as cohort studies [16,17] or historical controls [18]. It is difficult to make firm conclusions about the place of CPAP from these trials, not only because of design differences but to varying inclusion and intubation/extubation criteria.

Trials evaluating extubation to CPAP after mechanical ventilation have had mixed results. Annibale and colleagues [19] randomized infants of 600 to 1500 g birth weight to a brief period of nasopharyngeal CPAP, CPAP until resolution of lung disease, or head-box oxygen. Successful extubation did not vary among the three groups, even though about 70% received surfactant in all groups. In contrast, So and colleagues [20] randomized 50 infants less than 1500 g birth weight to nasal CPAP or oxygen hood and found significantly less need for reintubation in the nasal CPAP group. Higgins and colleagues [21] found similar results in infants less than 1000 g birth weight. Robertson and Hamilton [22] used the flow driver and randomized 58 babies to head-box oxygen or nasal CPAP. Nearly 100% of their babies received surfactant and mean birthweight was approximately 1000 g. No differences in ventilator days were found. Davis and colleagues [23] randomly assigned 92 infants of 600 to 1250 g birth weight to nasal CPAP or oxygen head box and reported 66% of nasal CPAP infants were successfully extubated compared with 40% of those treated with head-box oxygen.

A Cochrane review of NCPAP after extubation included a total of eight trials, in which 629 infants were treated in randomized or quasi-randomized trials of CPAP. Although there is significant heterogeneity for many of the outcomes, the review concluded that NCPAP is effective in preventing extubation failure [24]. After excluding one quasi-randomized trial, which contributed much of the heterogeneity, the relative risk (RR) for extubation failure when treated with CPAP rather than spontaneous ventilation was 0.57, 95% confidence intervals (0.46, 0.72). The absolute risk difference is 0.2, meaning that the number needed to treat with CPAP to prevent one extubation failure is only 5.

Continuous positive airway pressure device comparisons

There are few comparisons of different CPAP devices. The variable flow driver devices seem to function similarly to each other [25] and have been shown to recruit lung volume very effectively and to decrease work of breathing in the low birth weight infant (Figs. 3 and 4) [26,27]. In an infant study comparing rate of extubation failure, however, the variable flow device did not result in fewer reintubations [28]. Nonetheless, in infants receiving variable flow the oxygen requirement and length of stay were less than with conventional, continuous flow CPAP. In a similar but smaller study, Mazzella and colleagues [29] found lower oxygen requirements and respiratory rates in infants randomized to the flow driver compared with bubble CPAP delivered by a single hypopharyngeal prong.

Davis and colleagues [30] studied single versus binasal prongs in 87 infants less than 1000 g birth weight. Infants randomized to binasal prongs were more likely to be successfully extubated (76% versus 43%). This group also found short double prongs to have the lowest resistance to airflow when tested in a bench study [31].

The resurgence of bubble CPAP as a method of providing positive pressure largely results from its use at a single medical center, which reported less chronic lung disease than many other centers [32]. Bubble CPAP is an inexpensive method of providing CPAP. As applied to newborn infants, however, it does not act as a pure threshold (flow-independent) resistor,

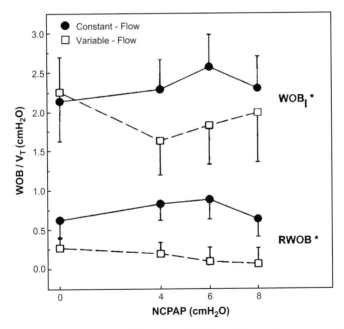

Fig. 3. Changes in inspiratory work of breathing (WOB_I) and the resistive component (RWOB) between constant and variable flow NCPAP (means ± SE). Overall, WOB_I and RWOB were significantly lower with the variable flow device (*$P < .001$). (*From* Pandit PB, Courtney SE, Pyon KH, el al. Work of breathing during constant- and variable-flow nasal continuous positive airway pressure in preterm neonates. Pediatrics 2001;108:682–5; with permission.)

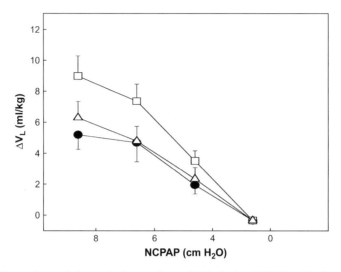

Fig. 4. Comparison of change in lung volume (ΔV_L) during NCPAP with three devices. Squares, variable flow NCPAP; triangles, constant flow NCPAP (6 LPM); circles, nasal cannula (6 LPM) (means ± SE). $P < .001$ variable flow versus both constant flow and nasal cannula. (*Modified from* Courtney SE, Pyon KH, Saslow JG, et al. Lung recruitment and breathing pattern during variable versus continuous flow nasal continuous positive airway pressure in premature infants: an evaluation of three devices. Pediatrics 2001;107:304–8; with permission.)

nor does it have the adjustable orifice size of a flow resistor [33]. In fact, flow can dramatically affect the delivered CPAP (Fig. 5), even in the presence of some leak at the nares. Because of this, measurement of pressure at the prongs is essential during use of bubble CPAP to prevent overdistension of the lungs. Some have argued that the oscillations provided by bubble CPAP may improve gas exchange [34]; however, others dispute this [35], and the marked attenuation of the waveform at the level of the alveoli makes this unlikely (Fig. 6). Liptsen and colleagues [36] have reported increased work of breathing with bubble CPAP compared with variable flow CPAP.

Nasal cannula continuous positive airway pressure

Several studies have shown that nasal cannula CPAP generation is possible [27,37,38]. How much depends on the flow rate, the size of the cannula prongs, the size of the infant, and the configuration of the airway.

Locke and coworkers [37] showed in a group of infants of about 1400 g birth weight that infant cannulas with external diameter of 0.3 cm could provide positive pressure at virtually any flow, with clinically significant positive pressure at flows of 1 to 2 liters per minute (LPM) —about 4–9 cm H_2O— and significant variability; at 2 LPM the mean plus 2 SD of esophageal pressure was greater than 15 cm H_2O. This finding was confirmed by Sreenan and colleagues [38], who provided a formula to approximate 6 cm H_2O using a nasal cannula in preterm infants. Courtney and colleagues [27]

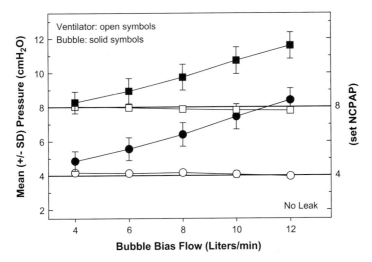

Fig. 5. In vitro study of NCPAP generated with a bubble system (*solid symbols*) and an infant ventilator under no-leak conditions. Set NCPAP levels of 4 and 8 cm H_2O, shown on the right-hand Y-axis, were maintained constant with the ventilator despite increasing flow levels. With the bubble system, increasing flow resulted in dramatic increases in NCPAP pressure as measured at the prongs. (*Courtesy of* Doron Kahn, MD, New Hyde Park, NY.)

found that an infant cannula used at 6 LPM could recruit lung volume equally well to a conventional continuous flow nasal CPAP device.

Recently, high-flow nasal cannula devices have been advertised as potential alternatives to CPAP. There is appropriate concern, however, that these devices cannot estimate actual CPAP delivered, nor is there a "pop-off" to prevent delivery of excessive pressure [39]. Additionally, higher pressures may occur than with either CPAP or a conventional cannula at similar flows [40]. Given that we have many devices available that can approximate airway pressure by measurement at the prongs, and that unknown, uncontrolled pressure is a potential danger in infants, it seems reasonable to relegate cannula use to low flow (<2 LPM), at which generation of significant positive pressure is unlikely. The American Association of Respiratory Care also recommends this practice [41].

Noninvasive ventilation

There has recently been substantial interest in the use of noninvasive methods of providing assisted ventilation. We define such methods as any mode of assisted ventilation that delivers positive pressure throughout the respiratory cycle with additional phasic increases in airway pressure, without the presence of an endotracheal tube. These additional phasic increases in airway pressure can be either synchronized to the infant's respiratory effort or nonsynchronized depending on the delivery system used.

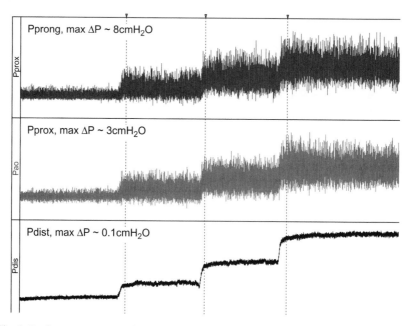

Fig. 6. In vitro measurement of prong (*Pprong*), proximal (*Pprox*), and distal (*Pdist*) pressures during bubble NCPAP at increasing bias flows (4, 6, 8, 10 L/minute) under small-leak conditions. Note the change in pressure amplitude from approximately 8 cm H_2O at the prongs to about 0.1 cm H_2O at the distal airway. (Not to scale.) (*Courtesy of* Sherry Courtney, MD, MS, New Hyde Park, NY.)

The terminology surrounding noninvasive ventilation is confusing. Some of the more common terms include NV (nasal ventilation), NIMV, SNIMV (synchronized nasal intermittent mandatory ventilation), NPSIMV (nasopharyngeal synchronized intermittent mandatory ventilation), and NPPV (non invasive positive pressure ventilation). Bilevel CPAP (BiPAP) also fits the definition, because it provides a phasic increase in pressure [42].

NIV provides the benefits of CPAP with the addition of positive pressure breaths. As noted above, CPAP splints the airway throughout the respiratory cycle, increases functional residual capacity, provides effective chest wall stabilization, improves ventilation perfusion mismatch, and thereby improves oxygenation. Studies of the physiologic effects of NIV have focused on synchronized modes. Compared with CPAP, synchronized NIV delivers larger tidal volumes by enhancing the transpulmonary pressure during inspiration, and also probably secondary to augmented inspiratory reflexes and sigh breaths [43]. Synchronized NIV leads to a reduction in respiratory rate, seems to decrease respiratory effort, and presumably (by increasing tidal volume) leads to a reduction in $Paco_2$. It also provides enhanced chest wall stabilization as evidenced by decreased asynchronous thoracoabdominal motion [44]. The increased peak transpulmonary pressures may further recruit atelectatic terminal air spaces. The physiologic effects of nonsynchronized NIV have not been studied in detail, but may actually trigger respiratory efforts by the Head's paradoxical reflex and provide assisted ventilation during apneic spells, as long as the airway is patent. Airway closure is known to occur during central and obstructive apnea, and the administration of sufficient positive expiratory pressure to maintain airway patency may be important. If the airway is patent during apnea, the positive pressure breaths during apnea may be sufficient to move the chest and thus reduce or prevent desaturation and bradycardia (Fig. 7, showing respiratory impedance deflections during an apnea while an infant is receiving NIV). Fig. 8 shows a similar apneic episode 1.5 hours later in the same patient while on nasal CPAP. A rapid and significant fall in saturation occurs, along with bradycardia. This observation requires further investigation.

Airflow can be delivered by way of binasal prongs, or a single prong placed with the tip in the nose or nasopharynx. Use of a face mask held in place by a device or netting around the head is not recommended, as it has been associated with cerebellar hemorrhage [45]. Newer nasal masks are now available, requiring less pressure to remain in place, but they must also be shown to be safe.

Nonsynchronized nasal ventilation can be delivered by any ventilator type. Synchronized nasal ventilation can only be delivered by respirators with specific triggering devices. These triggering devices have included body surface sensors, such as an abdominal pressure capsule or airflow

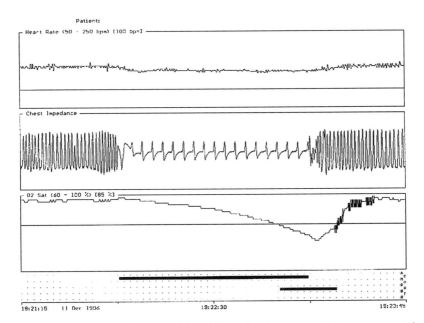

Fig. 7. Apnea in a preterm infant receiving NIV. During the apnea, which commences at the time of the abrupt change in the chest impedance pattern and lasts 70 seconds, there is no change in heart rate and saturation falls to 77%. (*Courtesy of* Keith Barrington, MD, Quebec, Canada.)

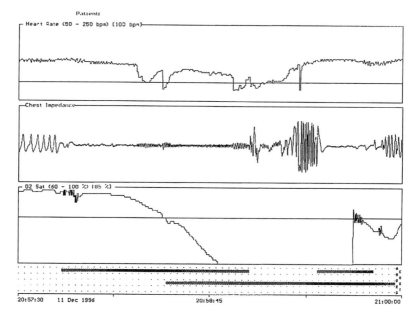

Fig. 8. Apnea in a preterm infant receiving CPAP. This is the same infant as Fig. 7; the apnea occurred approximately 1.5 hours after that recording. The first part of the apnea lasted 93 seconds, the infant became bradycardic after 35 seconds, and the saturation was below 60% after 70 seconds. (*Courtesy of* Keith Barrington, MD, Quebec, Canada.)

sensor [43]. The latter system was used in a short-term study and analyzes the flow from the sensor to eliminate flow resulting from oral or nasal leaks; thus the variation in the signal is related only to the patient's inspiration. In contrast, we have been unsuccessful in synchronizing NIV using flow sensors, because the leaks are huge and very variable, leading to great difficulty in detecting the patient's respiratory effort even in the short term.

Bilevel continuous positive airway pressure

BiPAP systems have been used in older patients and adults for years. Recent studies suggest that bilevel CPAP may be effective in avoiding intubation in some situations in older children. [46,47]. These systems cycle between two levels of positive pressure, and, as in other forms of noninvasive ventilation, allow patient breathing throughout the respiratory cycle. They are normally used with patient triggering of the inspiratory phase. There is little conceptual difference between BiPAP and other forms of NIV. BiPAP systems can be used with a much longer duration of the higher pressure plateau (>1 second); however, this is unstudied in small infants and must be shown to be safe.

A variable flow CPAP system with an abdominal wall sensor for breath synchronization is now available for use in neonates in Canada and Europe, and is referred to as a BiPAP system. One recent trial found improved oxygenation and ventilation during BiPAP use in low birth weight infants compared with CPAP [42]. In that trial, the inspiratory phase had a duration of 0.5 seconds and pressure of 4 cm H_2O above the expiratory pressure, making the system identical to NIV but with a lower-than-usual peak pressure. The current BiPAP device available for neonates uses variable flow technology. Given the improved recruitment capability of variable flow, it is prudent to avoid high levels of pressure when variable flow BiPAP is used to avoid overdistension of the lungs. Studies are needed to define the benefits and potential risks of BiPAP when it is used in the preterm infant.

Clinical trials of noninvasive ventilation

Postextubation

Three randomized controlled trials have demonstrated the efficacy of nasal IMV (all synchronized devices in these studies) compared with CPAP in reducing the need for reintubation following extubation [48–50]. A further randomized short-term crossover study referred to earlier [43] suggested that these benefits result from enhanced minute ventilation with reduced patient effort. A meta-analysis of the three trials revealed that the number needed to treat with nasal intermittent positive pressure ventilation is 3 to prevent one extubation failure, compared with postextubation use of CPAP [49].

Apnea of prematurity

Two studies have compared CPAP with NIMV (both nonsynchronized) specifically for the treatment of apnea of prematurity [50,51]. Both of these were short-term crossover studies (over 4 to 6 hours) and the results are conflicting. It is not clear whether NIMV reduces the frequency of apnea more effectively than NCPAP. In the postextubation studies noted above there was a trend toward a reduction in apnea frequency postextubation with NIMV compared with CPAP [49].

Using noninvasive ventilation

The settings chosen depend on the indication for assisted ventilation. Our postextubation study commenced with a PEEP of 6 cm H_2O and a peak inspiratory pressure to a maximum of 16 cm H_2O [48]. At these settings we did not see an increase in abdominal distension or feeding intolerance compared with CPAP alone. Individual patients may require higher PEEP (up to 7–8 cm H_2O on occasion). We generally start with a respiratory rate of 15 and an inspiratory time of 0.4 seconds.

The settings we choose for apnea of prematurity in the absence of significant lung disease are generally lower. When the pulmonary status is normal, NIV may be effective at a peak inspiratory pressure of 10 to 12 cm H_2O

and a PEEP between 4 and 6 cm H_2O. Higher PEEP may be required to prevent airway closure during apnea in some infants.

Clinicians must remember that as of this writing the only proven benefit of NIV compared with CPAP is a reduction in the need for reintubation during the first 72 hours after extubation of very low birth weight infants, using NIV devices that synchronize with the baby's inspiratory effort.

Continuous positive airway pressure: unresolved issues

Continuous positive airway pressure in the delivery room

Use of positive pressure in the delivery room makes theoretic sense. Establishing functional residual capacity quickly, thereby diminishing the potential lung damage from atelectrauma, is supported by animal data [52–54] and by human data outside of the delivery room as already discussed. Given that CPAP is used routinely in the NICU for infants who have mild or moderate respiratory distress, its use in the delivery room for the same infants is reasonable. Using CPAP in very immature babies who do not have respiratory distress, as a strategy against progressive lung derecruitment, is also frequent in the NICU, so starting it a few minutes earlier in the delivery room seems reasonable. A recent feasibility trial indicated that extremely low birth weight preterm infants could be randomized into a trial assessing use of CPAP in the delivery room [55]. Until a large, randomized, controlled trial is performed supporting this intervention, though, CPAP in the delivery room remains an experimental therapy.

Continuous positive airway pressure and surfactant

More uncertain is how CPAP and surfactant should be used together. Should surfactant be given, then CPAP used? Should CPAP be given and surfactant used if infants fail CPAP? Should CPAP be used, surfactant given, and infants immediately extubated back to CPAP? Can surfactant be safely and effectively delivered by CPAP as an aerosol? Studies are ongoing that may help answer some of these important questions. Surfactant is probably the best-studied intervention in neonatology. We know surfactant works and can reduce mortality significantly. The infant population of today is different from the years of the surfactant trials, however, predominantly because the use of prenatal steroids has increased dramatically. Until we have answers from ongoing trials, we would do well to use surfactant in infants who will benefit from it, and await the results of studies in progress.

Nasal intermittent mandatory ventilation: unresolved issues

Several key technical and clinical issues still need to be addressed. Is synchronization a necessary requirement for this form of respiratory support, and if so can we improve these systems to deliver synchronous breaths?

Noninvasive ventilation as a primary mode of treatment of respiratory distress syndrome?

There are no randomized studies addressing this mode of ventilation as a primary therapeutic intervention for the treatment of mild RDS and as such the routine use of NIMV for the treatment of RDS cannot be recommended at present. A short-term crossover study [56] compared physiologic responses to NIV and CPAP in preterm infants who had mild respiratory distress, at a postnatal age of 1 to 14 days. Six of these infants had previously been ventilated. This study confirmed that synchronized NIV significantly reduced the work of breathing compared with CPAP, when the peak applied pressure did not exceed 14 cm H_2O. Future studies addressing this use are warranted.

A prospective observational pilot study in preterm infants after surfactant treatment of RDS suggested that short-term respiratory outcomes might be improved by immediate extubation to NIV rather than by continuing intubation for a more conventional weaning period over an average of 2.4 days. The authors concluded that this might lead to other benefits, such as shorter hospitalization [57].

Noninvasive ventilation for apnea?

Some infants who have severe apnea and an inadequate response to other therapies, and who are intubated, develop significant chronic lung disease and other complications of prematurity. NIV, as an alternative to reintubation, is an attractive possibility that needs to be investigated to determine whether clinically important outcomes can be improved.

Another potential benefit is a reduction in apnea frequency following extubation as mentioned above, and also a reduction in chronic lung disease. There was a trend toward a reduction in the incidence of chronic lung disease in the two studies included in the meta-analysis of postextubation NIV [49] that reported this outcome (RR 0.73, 95% confidence intervals 0.49, 1.07). This important possibility needs to be addressed in an adequately powered study with chronic lung disease as a primary endpoint. Avoidance of endotracheal tube placement or a reduction in the duration of endotracheal intubation may also result in a reduction in the risk for airway injury and nosocomial respiratory infections; these possibilities also need further assessment.

Complications of continuous positive airway pressure and noninvasive ventilation

CPAP use has had few complications. Over- or underdistension of the lungs can occur if an inappropriate CPAP level is used. When using the variable flow driver devices that recruit lung better than conventional CPAP, clinicians must be vigilant to watch for overdistension [27].

CPAP devices, especially the prongs from the variable flow systems, have also been associated with necrosis of the nasal septum if the prongs are not placed properly in the nares [58]. Other forms of nasal erosion resulting from the prongs or facemask are potential risks, but with increasing experience using noninvasive forms of ventilatory support and good nursing care, serious nasal injury has become rare. Prongs less likely to cause this problem are being developed and will soon be available.

Gaseous distension of the abdomen (CPAP belly) occurs in some infants. Feeding intolerance or vomiting may occur. Infants having this problem often respond to a somewhat lower CPAP pressure or to continuous rather than bolus feedings. Transpyloric feeding is also an option. Although there are concerns regarding abdominal distension secondary to flow delivered preferentially to the stomach, the risk has not been reported to be higher with NIV than with CPAP in the randomized trials. These trials were all, however, with synchronized NIV. The risk may be higher in nonsynchronized NIV, because airway pressure may increase when the glottis is closed.

Gastric perforation has previously been associated with the use of NIV in a case control study of 15 patients, for whom NIV was being used as primary therapy for severe RDS [59]. This study used a tight-fitting face mask and substantially higher pressures than are usually used at present. The five subsequent randomized trials totaling more than 230 patients have not reported gastric perforation as a complication. If NIV is to be used as a primary therapy in infants who have significant lung disease, however, ongoing surveillance for this complication is vital.

Pneumothorax and other air leaks may occur during CPAP and could theoretically be more common with the higher pressures of NIV, although none have been reported in the randomized studies to date.

When to intubate, when to extubate

Neither CPAP nor NIV can meet the needs of the infant patient in all circumstances. Unfortunately, when to intubate and when to extubate remain highly controversial. Given this uncertainty, the common sense approach seems reasonable. Severe acidosis affects cellular metabolism. Although respiratory acidosis may have benefits in the critically ill older child or adult [60], both low and high $Paco_2$ may be dangerous to the preterm infant [61]. Oxygen seems to be more toxic at lower concentrations than we were aware of several years ago [62]. A high work of breathing in an infant who has distress after extubation requires increased caloric expenditure and exhausts the infant; in contrast, the presence of an endotracheal tube in the airway may substantially increase airway resistance and work of breathing. Conversely, prolonged intubation carries risks of infection, mucociliary impairment, atelectasis, and lung injury. Decisions also depend on the underlying lung condition, neurologic status of the infant, and often many other factors. Until we have data demonstrating the safety of strategies such as permissive hypercapnia, however, a middle ground approach is preferable, in hopes to prevent unwanted and unknown deleterious side effects.

Summary

CPAP and forms of noninvasive mechanical ventilation are important tools for the neonatologist today. CPAP can recruit the lung and prevent or decrease apnea, thereby preventing or decreasing the need for intubation. Noninvasive positive pressure breaths seem to further extend the applicability of CPAP. Many questions remain as to which, if any, CPAP and NIV system is better and under what circumstances. We must diligently seek the answers to these questions and not assume we know what is best before the data are available. We would do well to follow the advice of William Silverman, who said, "Teach thy tongue to say 'I do not know,' and thou shall progress."

References

[1] Gregory GA, Kitterman JA, Phibbs RH, et al. Treatment of the idiopathic respiratory-distress syndrome with continuous positive airway pressure. N Engl J Med 1971;284(24): 1333–40.

[2] Kattwinkel J, Fleming D, Cha CC, et al. A device for administration of continuous positive airway pressure by the nasal route. Pediatrics 1973;52:131–4.

[3] Miller MJ, DiFiore JM, Strohl KP, et al. Effects of nasal CPAP on supraglottic and total pulmonary resistance in preterm infants. J Appl Physiol 1990;68(1):141–6.

[4] Benveniste D, Berg O, Pedersen JEP. A technique for delivery of continuous positive airway pressure to the neonate. J Pediatr 1976;88(6):1015–9.

[5] Moa G, Nilsson K, Zetterstrom H, et al. A new device for administration of nasal continuous positive airway pressure in the newborn: an experimental study. Crit Care Med 1988;16: 1238–42.

[6] Klausner JF, Lee AY, Hutchison AA. Decreased imposed work with a new nasal continuous positive airway pressure device. Pediatr Pulmonol 1996;22:188–94.

[7] DePaoli AG, Davis PG, Faber B, et al. Devices and pressure sources for administration of nasal continuous positive airway pressure (NCPAP) in preterm neonates. Cochrane Database Syst Rev 2002;3:CD002977.

[8] Subramaniam P, Henderson-Smart DJ, Davis PG. Prophylactic nasal continuous positive airways pressure for preventing morbidity and mortality in very preterm infants. Cochrane Database Syst Rev 2005;3:CD001243.

[9] O'Donnell C, Davis P, Morley C. Positive end-expiratory pressure for resuscitation of new-born infants at birth. Cochrane Database Syst Rev 2003;3:CD004341.

[10] Ho JJ, Subramaniam P, Henderson-Smart DJ, et al. Continuous distending pressure for respiratory distress syndrome in preterm infants. Cochrane Database Syst Rev 2002;2: CD002271.

[11] Ho JJ, Henderson-Smart DJ, Davis PG. Early versus delayed initiation of continuous distending pressure for respiratory distress syndrome in preterm infants. Cochrane Database Syst Rev 2002;2:CD002975.

[12] Krouskop RW, Brown EG, Sweet AY. The early use of continuous positive airway pressure in the treatment of idiopathic respiratory distress syndrome. J Pediatr 1975;87(2):263–7.

[13] Han VKM, Beverley DW, Clarson C, et al. Randomized controlled trial of very early continuous distending pressure in the management of preterm infants. Early Hum Dev 1987;15: 21–32.

[14] Verder H, Robertson B, Greisen G, et al. Surfactant therapy and nasal continuous positive airway pressure for newborns with respiratory distress syndrome. N Engl J Med 1994;331: 1051–5.

[15] Sandri F, Ancora G, Lanzoni A, et al. Prophylactic nasal continuous positive airways pressure in newborns of 28-31 weeks gestation: multicentre randomized controlled clinical trial. Arch Dis Child Fetal Neonatal Ed 2004;89:F394–8.

[16] Jonsson B, Katz-Salamon M, Faxelius G. Neonatal care of very-low-birth weight infants in special-care units and neonatal intensive-care units in Stockholm. Early nasal continuous positive airway pressure versus mechanical ventilation: gains and losses. Acta Paediatr Suppl 1997;419:4–10.

[17] Lindner W, Vofsbeck S, Hummler H, et al. Delivery room management of extremely low birth weight infants: spontaneous breathing or intubation? Pediatrics 1999;103(5): 961–7.

[18] Gitterman MK, Fusch C, Gitterman AR. Early nasal continuous positive airway pressure treatment reduces the need for intubation in very low birth weight infants. Eur J Pediatr 1997;156:384–8.

[19] Annibale DJ, Hulsey TC, Engstrom PC, et al. Randomized, controlled trial of nasopharyngeal continuous positive airway pressure in the extubation of very low birth weight infants. J Pediatr 1994;124:455–60.

[20] So BH, Tamura M, Mishina J, et al. Application of nasal continuous positive airway pressure to early extubation in very low birthweight infants. Arch Dis Child Fetal Neonatal Ed 1995;72:F191–3.

[21] Higgins RD, Richter SE, Davis JM. Nasal continuous positive airway pressure facilitates extubation of very low birth weight neonates. Pediatrics 1991;88(5):999–1003.

[22] Robertson NJ, Hamilton PA. Randomised trial of elective continuous positive airway pressure (CPAP) compared with rescue CPAP after extubation. Arch Dis Child Fetal Neonatal Ed 1998;79:F58–60.

[23] Davis P, Jankov R, Doyle L, et al. Randomised, controlled trial of nasal continuous positive airway pressure in the extubation of infants weighing 600-1250g. Arch Dis Child Fetal Neonatal Ed 1998;79:F54–7.

[24] Davis PG, Henderson-Smart DJ. Nasal continuous positive airway pressure immediately after extubation for preventing morbidity in preterm infants. Cochrane Database Syst Rev 2003;2:CD000143.

[25] Courtney SE, Aghai ZH, Saslow JG, et al. Changes in lung volume and work of breathing: a comparison of two variable-flow nasal continuous positive airway pressure devices in very low birth weight infants. Pediatr Pulmonol 2003;36:248–52.

[26] Pandit PB, Courtney SE, Pyon KH, et al. Work of breathing during constant- and variable-flow nasal continuous positive airway pressure in preterm neonates. Pediatrics 2001;108(3): 682–5.

[27] Courtney SE, Pyon KH, Saslow JG, et al. Lung recruitment and breathing pattern during variable versus continuous flow nasal continuous positive airway pressure in premature infants: an evaluation of three devices. Pediatrics 2001;107(2):304–8.

[28] Stefanescu BM, Murphy WP, Hansell BJ, et al. A randomized, controlled trial comparing two different continuous positive airway pressure systems for the successful extubation of extremely low birth weight infants. Pediatrics 2003;112(5):1031–8.

[29] Mazzella M, Bellini C, Calevo MG, et al. A randomized control study comparing the Infant Flow Driver with nasal continuous positive airway pressure in preterm infants. Arch Dis Child Fetal Neonatal Ed 2001;85:F86–90.

[30] Davis P, Davies M, Faber B. A randomized controlled trial of two methods of delivering nasal continuous positive airway pressure after extubation to infants weighing less than 1000 g: binasal (Hudson) versus single nasal prongs. Arch Dis Child Fetal Neonatal Ed 2001;85(2): F82–5.

[31] De Paoli AG, Morley CJ, Davis PG. In vitro comparison of nasal continuous positive airway pressure devices for neonates. Arch Dis Child Fetal Neonatal Ed 2002;86:F42–5.

[32] Avery ME, Tooley WH, Keller JB, et al. Is chronic lung disease in low-birth-weight infants preventable? A survey of eight centers. Pediatrics 1987;79:26–30.

[33] Christensen EF, Jensen RH, Schonemann NK, et al. Flow-dependent properties of positive expiratory pressure devices. Monaldi Arch Chest Dis 1995;50(2):150–3.

[34] Pillow JJ, Travadi JN, Bubble CPAP. Is the noise important? An in vitro study. Pediatr Res 2005;57:826–30.

[35] Morley CJ, Lau R, De Paoli A, et al. Nasal continuous positive airway pressure: does bubbling improve gas exchange? Arch Dis Child Fetal Neonatal Ed 2005;90:F343–4.

[36] Liptsen E, Aghai ZH, Pyon KH, et al. Work of breathing during nasal continuous positive airway pressure in preterm infants: a comparison of bubble vs variable-flow devices. J Perinatol 2005;25:453–8.

[37] Locke RC, Wolfson MR, Shaffer TH. Inadvertent administration of positive end-distending pressure during nasal cannula flow. Pediatrics 1993;91(1):135–8.

[38] Sreenan C, Lemke RP, Hudson-Mason A, et al. High-flow nasal cannulae in the management of apnea of prematurity: a comparison with conventional nasal continuous positive airway pressure. Pediatrics 2001;107(5):1081–3.

[39] Finer NN. Nasal cannula use in the preterm infant: oxygen or pressure? Pediatrics 2005; 116(5):1216–7.

[40] Chang GY, Cox CC, Shaffer TH. Nasal cannula, CPAP and vapotherm: effect of flow on temperature, humidity, pressure and resistance. PAS 2005;57:1231.

[41] American Association of Respiratory Care. AARC clinical practice guideline: selection of an oxygen delivery device for neonatal and pediatric patients – 2002 revision & update. Respir Care 2002;47:707–16.

[42] Migliori C, Motta M, Angeli A, et al. Nasal bilevel vs. continuous positive airway pressure in preterm infants. Pediatr Pulmonol 2005;40:426–30.

[43] Moretti C, Gizzi C, Papoff P, et al. Comparing the effects of nasal synchronized intermittent positive pressure ventilation (nSIPPV) and nasal continuous positive airway pressure (nCPAP) after extubation in very low birth weight infants. Early Hum Dev 1999;56:167–77.

[44] Kiciman NM, Andreasson B, Bernstein G, et al. Thoracoabdominal motion in newborns during ventilation delivered by endotracheal tube or nasal prongs. Pediatr Pulmonol 1998; 25:175–81.

[45] Pape KE, Armstrong DL, Fitzhardinge PM. Central nervous system pathology associated with mask ventilation in the very low birth weight infant: a new etiology for intracerebellar hemorrhages. Pediatrics 1976;58:473–83.

[46] Padman R, Lawless ST, Kettrick RG. Noninvasive ventilation via bilevel positive airway pressure support in pediatric practice. Crit Care Med 1998;26:169–73.

[47] Migliori C, Cavazza A, Motta M, et al. Early use of nasal-BiPAP in two infants with congenital central hypoventilation syndrome. Acta Paediatr 2003;92:823–6.

[48] Barrington KJ, Bull D, Finer NN. Randomized trial of nasal synchronized intermittent mandatory ventilation compared with continuous positive airway pressure after extubation of very low birth weight infants. Pediatrics 2001;107:638–41.

[49] Davis PG, Lemyre B, de Paoli AG. Nasal intermittent positive pressure ventilation (NIPPV) versus nasal continuous positive airway pressure (NCPAP) for preterm neonates after extubation. Cochrane Database Syst Rev 2001;3:CD003212.

[50] Ryan CA, Finer NN, Peters KL. Nasal intermittent positive-pressure ventilation offers no advantages over nasal continuous positive airway pressure in apnea of prematurity. Am J Dis Child 1989;143(10):1196–8.

[51] Lin CH, Wang ST, Lin YJ, et al. Efficacy of nasal intermittent positive pressure ventilation in treating apnea of prematurity. Pediatr Pulmonol 1998;26(5):349–53.

[52] Naik AS, Kallapur SG, Bachurski CJ, et al. Effects of ventilation with different positive end-expiratory pressures on cytokine expression in the preterm lamb lung. Am J Respir Crit Care Med 2001;164:494–8.

[53] Mulrooney N, Champion Z, Moss TJM, et al. Surfactant and physiologic responses of preterm lambs to continuous positive airway pressure. Am J Respir Crit Care Med 2005;171: 488–93.

[54] Thomson MA, Yoder BA, Winter VT, et al. Treatment of immature baboons for 28 days with early nasal continuous positive airway pressure. Am J Respir Crit Care Med 2004; 169:1054–62.

[55] Finer NN, Carlo WA, Duara S, et al. Delivery room continuous positive airway pressure/ positive end-expiratory pressure in extremely low birth weight infants: a feasibility trial. Pediatrics 2004;114:651–65.

[56] Aghai ZH, Saslow JG, Nakhla T, et al. Synchronized nasal intermittent positive pressure ventilation (SNIPPV) decreases work of breathing (WOB) in premature infants with respiratory distress syndrome (RDS) compared to nasal continuous positive airway pressure (NCPAP). Pediatr Pulmonol 2006;41:875–81.

[57] Santin R, Brodsky N, Bhandari VA. A prospective observational pilot study of synchronized nasal intermittent positive airway pressure (SNIPPV) as a primary mode of ventilation in infants ≥28 weeks with respiratory distress syndrome (RDS). J Perinatol 2004;24:487–93.

[58] Yong S-C, Chen S-J, Boo N-Y. Incidence of nasal trauma associated with nasal prong versus nasal mask during continuous positive airway pressure treatment in very low birthweight infants: a randomised control study. Arch Dis Child Fetal Neonatal Ed 2005;90:F480–3.

[59] Garland JS, Nelson DB, Rice T, et al. Increased risk of gastrointestinal perforations in neonates mechanically ventilated with either face mask or nasal prongs. Pediatrics 1985; 76:406–10.

[60] Kregenow DA, Rubenfeld GD, Hudson LD, et al. Hypercapnic acidosis and mortality in acute lung injury. Crit Care Med 2006;34:1–7.

[61] Gressens P, Rogido M, Paindaveine B, et al. The impact of neonatal intensive care practices on the developing brain. J Pediatr 2002;140:646–53.

[62] Tin W, Wariyar U. Giving small babies oxygen: 50 years of uncertainty. Semin Neonatol 2002;7:361–7.

ELSEVIER
SAUNDERS

CLINICS IN
PERINATOLOGY

Clin Perinatol 34 (2007) 93–105

Volume-Targeted Ventilation of Newborns

Jaideep Singh, MD, MRCPCH[a], Sunil K. Sinha, MD, PhD, FRCP, FRCPCH[b],*, Steven M. Donn, MD[c]

[a]James Cook University Hospital, Marton Road, Middlesbrough, TS4 3BW, UK
[b]University of Durham and James Cook University Hospital, Marton Road, Middlesbrough, TS4 3BW, UK
[c]Division of Neonatal-Perinatal Medicine, C.S. Mott Children's Hospital, University of Michigan Health System, 1500 E. Medical Center Drive, Ann Arbor, MI 48109-0254, USA

Traditionally, neonatal ventilation has been accomplished using time-cycled pressure-limited ventilation (TCPLV), wherein the peak inspiratory pressure is selected by the clinician and the ventilator provides each breath without exceeding this set pressure. Because peak pressure was believed to be the primary determinant of lung injury through barotrauma, it was assumed that TCPLV would limit lung injury by its ability to control peak pressure. This is an oversimplification. From recent observations it seems that it may actually be the volume of gas delivered to the lungs that is more likely to be the primary determinant of lung damage during mechanical ventilation [1]. This finding has given rise to the concept of volutrauma, which is fundamental to understanding the concept of lung volume-pressure hysteresis and the mechanisms of ventilator-induced lung injury (VILI) [2]. It has been shown in animal models that only six manual inflations of 35 to 40 mL/kg given to preterm lambs injures lungs and reduces the response to surfactant therapy [3]. Dreyfuss and colleagues [4] observed significant increases in lung edema and transcapillary albumin flux in rats ventilated at high tidal volumes in contrast to rats ventilated with low tidal volumes and high pressures. In another study, high-pressure ventilation with high tidal volumes caused a sevenfold increase in lung lymph flow and protein clearance in sheep, whereas high pressure ventilation with a normal tidal

Dr. Singh's work was supported by a NHS Research & Development Grant.
Dr. Donn serves on the Clinical Advisory Board, is a consultant, and is a member of the Speakers Bureau of Viasys Healthcare, Inc.
* Corresponding author.
E-mail address: sunil.sinha@stees.nhs.uk (S.K. Sinha).

doi:10.1016/j.clp.2006.12.007   *perinatology.theclinics.com*

volume obtained by chest strapping produced a 35% decrease in lymph flow and protein clearance [5]. Hernandez and colleagues [6] could completely block microvascular damage in ventilated rabbit lungs using tidal volume limitation. Evidence for the importance of volutrauma also comes from the adult acute respiratory distress syndrome network trial [7]. Traditional approaches to mechanical ventilation in adults used tidal volumes of 10 to 15 mL/kg in patients who had acute lung injury and acute respiratory distress syndrome. This trial was conducted to determine whether ventilation with lower tidal volumes would improve the clinical outcomes in these patients. The trial found that using lower tidal volumes decreased mortality and increased the number of days without ventilator use.

Conversely, ventilation at low lung volumes may also cause lung injury, especially in surfactant-deficient lungs. This injury is believed to be related to the repeated opening and closing of lung units with each mechanical breath (atelectotrauma). This phenomenon may explain the observation that recruitment of lung to increase the functional residual capacity protects against VILI [8,9].

If volutrauma is indeed important in the development of VILI then volume-controlled ventilation (VCV) may have advantages over TCPLV.

One of the first ventilators designed and built specifically for use in infants was a volume-controlled device. This version was eventually discarded because of technological limitations, including long response times, an ineffective triggering system, inability to deliver the small tidal volumes needed by preterm newborns, a highly compliant circuit (which increased compressible volume loss), and a lack of continuous flow during spontaneous breathing. Since the introduction of microprocessor-based ventilators, however, it is now possible toventilate even the smallest of babies using VCV. This use has been facilitated by the development of sensitive and accurate flow sensors and servo-controlled mechanics allowing accurate measurement and tracking of gas flow to avoid overexpansion (volutrauma) or underexpansion (atelectotrauma) of the lungs and damage attributable to airway flow that is too high or too low (rheotrauma). This development may have advantages particularly in newborns who have respiratory distress syndrome (RDS) in whom lung compliance (and hence delivery of gas volume to the lungs) may rapidly change in response to the disease process or treatment, such as surfactant therapy.

VCV differs from volume guarantee (VG), pressure-regulated volume control (PRVC) or volume-assured pressure support (VAPS), which are hybrid forms of ventilation (see related articles in this issue). These are essentially pressure-limited modes of ventilation that use dual loop control to maintain tidal volume delivery in the target range. These newer forms of ventilation often lead to confusion and it is crucial that clinicians familiarize themselves with the new nomenclature and differences among them, which are often specific to individual devices.

Principles of time-cycled pressure-limited ventilation and volume-controlled ventilation

How does VCV differ from TCPLV? The difference was elegantly described by Carlo and colleagues [10]. Ventilators can be classified by the variables that are controlled (pressure, volume, or flow, which is the integral of volume), and the phase variables, such as those that start (trigger), sustain (or limit), and end (cycle) inspiration. At any one time, a ventilator can be only pressure controlled or volume controlled. Pressure- and volume-controlled breath types have certain specific characteristics, which are retained even if changes are made in phase variables by altering the trigger, limit, or cycling mechanism. For example, in TCPLV, a peak inspiratory pressure is set by the operator, and during inspiration gas flow is delivered to achieve that target pressure. The volume of gas delivered to the patient, however, is variable depending on the compliance of the lungs. At lower compliance (such as early in the course of RDS), a given pressure generates lower tidal volume compared with later in the course of the disease when the lungs are more compliant. This phenomenon is illustrated in Fig. 1a.

In contrast, the key differentiating feature of VCV is that the primary gas delivery target is tidal volume, which is set by the operator, and the peak inspiratory pressure may vary from breath to breath. At lower compliance higher pressures are generated to deliver the set tidal volume. As compliance improves, the pressure needed to achieve the set tidal volume is automatically reduced (auto-weaning of pressure). This relationship is illustrated in Fig. 1b.

In adult VCV inspiration is terminated and the machine is cycled into expiration when the target tidal volume is delivered. This process gave rise to the term "volume-cycled ventilation." The use of uncuffed endotracheal tubes in newborns results in some degree of gas leak around the tube, however. True volume cycling thus is a misnomer in neonatal ventilation and the terms volume controlled, volume targeted, or volume limited better describe this modality [11]. Most modern ventilators provide the option of using a leak compensation algorithm to offset this problem. One should also realize that there is a discrepancy between the volume of gas leaving the ventilator and that reaching the proximal airway. Much of this results from compression of gas within the ventilator circuit. This phenomenon is referred to as compressible volume loss. It is greatest when pulmonary compliance is lowest. Use of semi-rigid circuits may help to minimize this. It is also affected by humidification. It is therefore critical to measure the delivered tidal volume as close to the patient as possible (ie, at the patient wye piece). Most current ventilators measure volume delivery during inspiration (V_{Ti}) and expiration (V_{Te}). This measurement also enables quantification of gas leak and accurate compensation.

Another important feature of VCV differentiating it from TCPLV is the way that gas is delivered during inspiration. In traditional VCV, a square flow waveform is generated (Fig. 2) and peak volume delivery is achieved

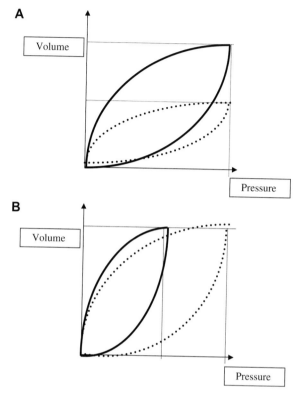

Fig. 1. (*A*) Pressure-volume loops in pressure-limited ventilation. Pressure is plotted on horizontal axis and tidal volume delivered on vertical axis. In low compliance lung (broken line
loop) the tidal volume delivered is lower than compliant lung (continuous line loop). Pressure
delivered by the ventilator is same for the two breaths. (*B*) Pressure-volume loops in volume-
controlled ventilation. Pressure is plotted on horizontal axis and tidal volume delivered on vertical axis. Tidal volume delivered is same for the two breaths. In low compliance lung (broken
line loop) the pressure needed to deliver the set tidal volume is higher than in compliant lung
(continuous line loop).

at the end of inspiration [11]. Newer ventilators do allow the option of
choosing a decelerating flow waveform. During VCV, inspiratory time is determined by the inspiratory flow rate. Because higher flow rates lead to more
rapid filling of the lungs, set tidal volumes are achieved faster, which leads to
an inverse relationship between flow and inspiratory time in VCV. In contrast, during TCPLV flow is sinusoidal and the opening pressure is reached
quickly (see Fig. 2). After the target pressure has been reached, flow decelerates rapidly until inspiration is complete. The fixed inspiratory time allows
more time for the alveoli to fill giving a theoretical advantage if high opening pressures are necessary, such as during the acute stages of RDS.

As with TCPLV, VCV can be provided in various modes, including intermittent mandatory ventilation (IMV), synchronized intermittent mandatory

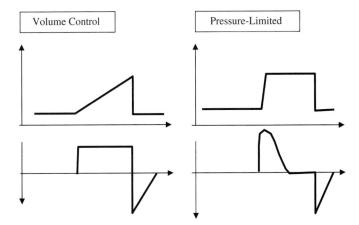

Fig. 2. Pressure and flow waveforms illustrate the difference between volume-control and pressure-limited ventilation. The upper panel represents pressure waveform and the lower panel flow waveform. Volume-control waveforms are shown on the left and pressure-limited on the right.

ventilation (SIMV), and assist/control ventilation (A/C) (Fig. 3). It may also be combined with pressure support ventilation (PSV) during SIMV.

Hybrid ventilation

Because TCPLV and VCV have specific advantages and disadvantages (Box 1), combined or hybrid forms of ventilation have been developed in an attempt to combine the best features of each. These are primarily pressure-limited types of ventilation, but the delivered tidal volume is continuously monitored by the ventilator, and if it is less than the desired level, the peak pressure setting or inspiratory time are automatically adjusted to optimize tidal volume delivery. The available hybrid forms include VG, PRVC, and VAPS.

Volume guarantee ventilation

VG is a combined ventilator modality perhaps best described as a double or dual loop synchronized modality that ventilates using TCPL breaths with continuous flow, but it allows the pressure to be adjusted up to a clinician-set maximum using microprocessor technology to guarantee tidal volume delivery. The auto-feedback method, based on the previous breaths, aims to guarantee tidal volume delivery within a set range. The starting tidal volume target is usually 4 to 6 mL/kg. The maximum pressure limit is usually set about 20% greater than the pressure needed to deliver this tidal volume consistently. VG allows the clinician control of maximum airway pressure but also allows the ventilator to make appropriate adjustments of the

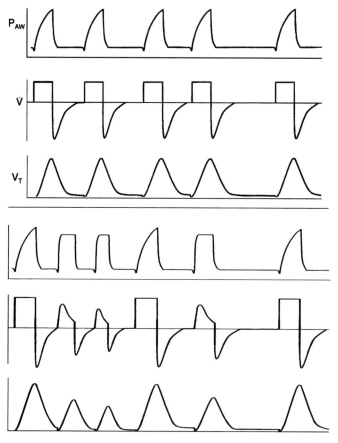

Fig. 3. Graphic waveforms. Upper panel demonstrates pressure, flow, and volume waveforms during volume-controlled assist/control. Note the square flow waveform and consistent tidal volume delivery. Lower panel demonstrates pressure, flow, and volume waveforms during volume-controlled synchronized intermittent mandatory ventilation (SIMV) with pressure support (PS). SIMV breaths are recognizable by square flow waveform and "shark's fin" pressure waveform, whereas PS breaths show a sinusoidal flow waveform.

peak airway pressure up to the set maximum to achieve the set tidal volume. The peak pressure achieved by the ventilator thus varies between the baseline pressure (PEEP) and the set peak inspiratory pressure (PIP). Potential advantages of VG include (1) less risk for volutrauma, because the clinician can limit tidal volume delivery; (2) reduced peak pressure, such as when the baby makes a significant contribution from spontaneous effort; (3) more stable tidal volume delivery; and (4) auto-weaning of peak inspiratory pressure, which may reduce barotrauma. Clinicians using VG should be aware of limitations associated with the feedback loop mechanism, however, and must be willing to make necessary adjustments to minimize potential harm. For example, as adjustments to PIP are made in small increments to avoid

---

Box 1. Perceived advantages and disadvantages of volume-controlled and pressure-limited ventilation

Volume-controlled ventilation
Constant tidal volume delivery even with varying pulmonary compliance
Linear increase in minute volume delivery as tidal volume increases
Excessive peak pressure could increase barotraumas
Auto-weaning of airway pressure as lung compliance improves

Time-cycled pressure-limited ventilation
Limits peak airway pressure and thus limits barotrauma
Improves gas distribution as set PIP is achieved throughout inspiratory cycle
Reduces work of breathing by providing high initial flow
Variable tidal volume delivery–risk for high tidal volume delivery as compliance improves or inadequate delivery if compliance worsens unless manually adjusted

---

Abbreviation: PIP, peak inspiratory pressure.

---

overcompensation, the delivered tidal volume may not compensate for large breath-to-breath fluctuations. Although VG leads to more consistent tidal volume delivery, this may not always be the actual set tidal volume. Moreover, because variation in pressure is based on the exhaled tidal volume of the previous breath, it does not truly make real time adjustments. In the presence of large endotracheal tube leaks, it may underestimate tidal volume delivery and overcompensate on subsequent breaths. To date, however, three small published studies have not shown any harm in using VG [12–16].

Pressure-regulated volume control

PRVC is another hybrid form of ventilation. It is flow-cycled and offers the variable flow rate of pressure-control ventilation with the additional benefit of a targeted tidal volume. PRVC is also a form of closed-loop ventilation, in which pressure is adjusted according to the delivered tidal volume. The clinician sets a target tidal volume and the maximum pressure. The first breath is a VC breath and is used as a test breath to enable the microprocessor to calculate the pressure needed to deliver the set tidal volume based on the patient's compliance. The next breaths are of variable flow. The mode therefore produces the same pressure and flow patterns as pressure control but also targets tidal volume delivered on each breath and adjusts the PIP on the subsequent breath.

PRVC provides the benefits of pressure-limited ventilation (maximum pressure set by the clinician) with guarantee of set tidal volume delivery. The ventilator allows the delivery of PRVC with other modalities (pressure-controlled and volume-controlled ventilation) called "automode," which allows the patient to breathe spontaneously while guaranteeing volume with pressure support and providing control ventilation in case of poor patient respiratory drive. A proximal flow transducer has also been introduced.

Volume-assured pressure support ventilation

VAPS is an unusual hybrid form in that it combines volume- and pressure-targeted ventilation within a single breath, rather than using a breath-averaging algorithm. VAPS can best be described as variable flow volume ventilation, which blends PSV and VCV. Each breath starts as a variable flow pressure support breath. The ventilator measures the delivered tidal volume when the inspiratory flow has decelerated to a minimum set level. If the delivered tidal volume equals or exceeds the desired tidal volume, the breath continues and then terminates as a typical flow-cycled pressure support breath. If the targeted tidal volume is not achieved, the breath transitions to a VCV breath by prolonging the inspiratory time (which can be limited) and slightly ramping up the pressure until the set tidal volume is delivered. Little clinical information on the neonatal applications of VAPS exists, but it may be advantageous in situations in which there is either rapidly changing compliance or erratic spontaneous respiratory drive.

Clinical studies

Compared with TCPLV, VCV is relatively new to the neonatal intensive care unit. There are not many controlled studies describing its safety and efficacy, although most published trials are favorable.

In a recent Cochrane review, McCallion and colleagues [17] identified eight randomized trials comparing the use of volume-targeted versus traditional pressure-limited ventilation in neonates. Only four met the eligibility criteria for inclusion in the meta-analysis. These four trials recruited a total of 178 preterm infants. The four trials are summarized below.

The first reported randomized controlled trial of true VCV versus TCPLV, which controlled tidal volume delivery in both arms of the trial, was conducted by Sinha and colleagues [18]. Fifty preterm infants weighing 1200 g or more who had RDS were randomly allocated to either VCV or TCPLV. Tidal volume delivery was set at 5 to 8 mL/kg in both groups so that the only difference was the ventilatory modality. The two groups were compared for the time required to achieve success criteria using the alveolar-arterial oxygen gradient (AaDo$_2$) or the mean airway pressure (Paw).

Infants randomized to VCV met the success criteria faster (mean time 65 versus 125 hours; $P < .001$) and had a shorter total duration of ventilation (mean time 122 versus 161 hours; $P < .001$). These babies also had a significantly lower incidence of large intraventricular hemorrhages and abnormal periventricular echodensities on ultrasound scans. There were no differences between the study groups in other complications associated with mechanical ventilation. Because of technological limitations in the minimum tidal volume delivery, infants weighing less than 1200 g could not be included in this first trial.

In another study performed contemporaneously, Piotrowski and colleagues [19] compared PRVC to traditional TCPL IMV. Sixty newborn babies weighing less than 2500 g and needing ventilation for RDS or congenital pneumonia were randomized to receive PRVC or IMV. The primary outcome measures were duration of mechanical ventilation and the incidence of CLD. Pulmonary air leaks and IVH were considered major adverse outcome measures. Duration of mechanical ventilation and incidence of CLD were similar in the two groups; however, the PRVC group had a lower incidence of Grade 2 IVH ($P < .05$) and fewer infants receiving PRVC had air leaks (3 versus 7). In a subgroup of infants weighing less than 1000 g, the duration of mechanical ventilation and incidence of hypotension were reduced in the PRVC group ($P < .05$).

The third study in this meta-analysis came from Keszler and Abubakar [12], who tested the hypothesis that VG would maintain the tidal volume and $PaCO_2$ within a target range more consistently than TCPLV used alone in the A/C mode. Eighteen preterm infants were randomized. VG significantly reduced the incidence of large tidal volume breaths (>6 mL/kg) more consistently but also significantly reduced the incidence of hypocarbia. They hypothesized that the use of VG had the potential to reduce the pulmonary and neurologic complications of mechanical ventilation.

On a similar theme, Lista and colleagues [14] evaluated the lung inflammatory response in preterm infants who had RDS, who were mechanically ventilated with and without VG, by measuring proinflammatory cytokines (IL-6, IL-8, TNF-α) in tracheobronchial aspirate fluid. Fifty-three preterm infants (gestational ages 25–32 weeks) were randomized to be ventilated using PSV with VG (tidal volume = 5 mL/kg) and PSV without VG. The trial found a significant difference in IL-8 and IL-6 levels on day 3 between the two groups. Infants who received PSV alone required 50% more ventilation (12.3 ± 3 versus 8.8 ± 3 days), although this difference was not statistically significant because of the small sample size.

These four trials included in the Cochrane review used different ventilators and techniques but shared the common aim of investigating the putative advantages of controlling tidal volume delivery in the optimal range among premature infants who required mechanical ventilation during the first 72 hours of life [17]. No significant difference was found for the primary outcome of death before discharge. None of the four trials reported the combined outcome of death or CLD. Analysis of the trials, however, showed that VCV resulted in a significant reduction in the duration of ventilation (weighted mean difference -2.93 days $[-4.28, -1.57]$) and the rate of pneumothorax (typical relative risk [RR] 0.23 [0.07, 0.76], risk difference [RD] -0.11 $[-0.20, -0.03]$, number needed to treat [NNT] 9). There was also a significant difference in the rate of severe (grade 3 or 4) intraventricular hemorrhage favoring VCV (typical RR 0.32 [0.11, 0.90], RD -0.16 $[-0.29, -0.03]$, NNT 6). There was a reduction in the incidence of BPD (supplemental oxygen at 36 weeks) among surviving infants, of borderline statistical significance (typical RR 0.34 [0.11, 1.05], RD -0.14 $[-0.27, 0.00]$, NNT 7). Long-term outcomes were not addressed.

Subsequently, technological refinements in one of the ventilators enabled performance of an additional randomized trial, this time enrolling even smaller preterm babies. Singh and colleagues [20] compared the safety and efficacy of VCV to TCPLV in very low birth weight infants who had respiratory failure at birth and required mechanical ventilation. The results are the most recent on this subject and should only strengthen the findings of the meta-analysis in support of VCV.

In this study, 109 newborns 24 to 31 weeks' gestation and weighing 600 to 1500 g at birth were randomized to receive either VCV or TCPLV. In both groups, ventilator variables were set to target an V_{Te} of 4 to 6 mL/kg monitored and adjusted on an hourly basis. In the VCV group, delivered tidal volume was adjusted, and in the TCPL group, the peak inspiratory pressure was adjusted. During the acute phase of illness, all infants were placed in the assist/control mode. Targeted blood gas indices, including a pH 7.25 to 7.40, $Paco_2$ 4.5 to 6.5 kPa (35–49 mm Hg), and Pao_2 7 to 10 kPa (50–75 mm Hg) were used during the initial stage. Subsequently, $Paco_2$ was permitted to increase to 8 kPa (60 mm Hg) if the pH remained greater than 7.20. Once the infants were recovering from acute illness (PIP < 16 cm H_2O and Fio_2 < 0.3), the ventilatory mode was changed to SIMV with PSV. The two modalities were compared by determining the time required to achieve either an $AaDo_2$ less than 100 mm Hg or a mean Paw less than 8 cm H_2O. Secondary outcomes included mortality, duration of mechanical ventilation, and complications associated with ventilation. The mean time to reach the success criterion was 23 hours with VCV versus 33 hours with TCPLV ($P = .15$). This difference, however, was more striking in babies weighing less than 1000 g (21 versus 58 hours; $P = .03$). Mean duration of ventilation with VCV was 255 hours versus 327 hours with TCPLV ($P = .60$). There was no significant difference in the incidence of complications between groups. All deaths in the first week of life were related to respiratory disease and occurred exclusively in infants randomized to TCPLV. This finding was unexpected, because the groups were closely matched for severity of RDS. Although the modality of ventilation did not show an independent effect on survival on multivariate analysis, there was a trend toward better survival among babies treated with VCV (odds ratio, 0.5; 95% CI,

0.2–1.2; $P = .10$). These findings should be interpreted with caution because of the sample size. One explanation for this difference might lie in the way in which flow (and hence volume) is delivered. During TCPLV there is rapid flow delivery, resulting in a sharp increase in airway pressure and delivery of volume early in the inspiratory phase. Theoretically, this should favor the expansion of the more compliant areas of the lung, possibly leading to nonhomogeneous gas delivery. In VCV, there is a slower but more sustained increase in inspiratory pressure, with peak volume delivery occurring at end-inspiration. This might result in more uniform filling of the lung and less atelectotrauma. A further benefit might accrue from auto-weaning. Although a similar tidal volume target was selected for both groups, changes in the TCPLV group required a clinical decision, which may not have been performed as rapidly.

Other studies have also looked at the efficacy of VCV. Weiswasser and colleagues [21] examined differences in pulmonary vascular resistance (PVR), cardiac index (CI), and dynamic compliance (Cdyn) in healthy and a surfactant-deficient neonatal piglet model. Animals were randomly assigned to VCV or TCPLV using perfluorocarbon liquid ventilation. Although there was no significant difference in healthy lungs, in the surfactant-deficient model Cdyn was significantly higher and PVR was significantly lower in the VCV group after 180 minutes of lung injury. Cardiac index declined significantly in both groups irrespective of ventilatory modality.

Hummler and colleagues [22] performed a crossover study to compare volume-controlled SIMV with pressure-limited SIMV in a population of 15 mechanically ventilated babies exhibiting frequent hypoxemic episodes. Although there was no significant difference between the two groups with respect to primary outcome measure (time with oxygen saturation <80%), babies randomized to volume SIMV maintained tidal volume better during episodes of desaturation, and bradycardia was less frequent in the volume SIMV group.

Summary

VCV and other volume-targeted modalities, such as VG, PRVC, and VAPS are new to neonatal intensive care and represent a departure from traditional TCPLV. Not surprisingly, there are only a few published randomized controlled clinical trials testing these modalities in the newborn population. Nonetheless, the evidence so far is highly encouraging. It seems that the consistency of tidal volume delivery during VCV in the face of varying lung compliance and the auto-weaning of airway pressure may be clinically advantageous, especially in conditions in which lung compliance can change rapidly, such as after surfactant treatment of RDS. Volume-targeted modalities have in common an objective to control tidal volume delivery in an attempt to provide optimal lung inflation. Stability of tidal volume delivery may be beneficial, especially in extremely low birth weight infants, who are at increased risk for sustaining complications associated with mechanical ventilation. Although the benefits of VCV in the published studies have been restricted to short-term outcomes, such as duration of ventilation, pneumothorax, and intraventricular hemorrhage, they are still important findings and should not be ignored. The preliminary trials also have laid the groundwork for larger multicenter trials of a sufficient size to be able to address the question of whether VCV improves the long-term respiratory and neurodevelopmental outcomes of preterm infants requiring mechanical ventilation [23].

References

[1] Dreyfuss D, Saumon G. Barotrauma is volutrauma, but which volume is the one responsible? Intensive Care Med 1992;18:139–41.

[2] Sinha S, Donn SM. Minimizing ventilator induced lung injury in preterm infants. Arch Dis Child Fetal Neonatal Ed 2006;91:F226–30.

[3] Bjorklund LJ, Ingimarsson J, Curstedt T, et al. Manual ventilation with a few large breaths at birth compromises the therapeutic effect of subsequent surfactant replacement in immature lambs. Pediatr Res 1997;42:348–55.

[4] Dreyfuss D, Soler P, Basset G, et al. High inflation pressure pulmonary edema. Respective effects of high airway pressure, high tidal volume, and positive end-expiratory pressure. Am Rev Respir Dis 1988;137:1159–64.

[5] Carlton D, Cummings JJ, Scheerer R, et al. Lung overexpansion increases pulmonary microvascular protein permeability in young lambs. J Appl Physiol 1990;69:577–83.

[6] Hernandez L, Peevy K, Moise A, et al. Chest wall restriction limits high airway pressure-induced injury in young rabbits. J Appl Physiol 1989;66:2364–8.

[7] Anon. Ventilation with lower tidal volumes as compared with traditional tidal volumes for acute lung injury and the acute respiratory distress syndrome. The Acute Respiratory Distress Syndrome Network. N Engl J Med 2000;342:1301–8.

[8] McCulloch PR, Forkert PG, Froese AB. Lung volume maintenance prevents lung injury during high frequency oscillatory ventilation in surfactant-deficient rabbits. Am Rev Respir Dis 1988;137:1185–92.

[9] Dreyfuss D, Saumon G. Role of tidal volume, FRC, and end-inspiratory volume in the development of pulmonary edema following mechanical ventilation. Am Rev Respir Dis 1993;148:1194–203.

[10] Carlo WA, Ambalavanan N, Chatburn RL. Classification of mechanical ventilation devices. In: Donn S, Sinha SK, editors. Manual of neonatal respiratory care. 2nd edition. Philadelphia: Mosby Elsevier; 2006. p. 74–80.

[11] Sinha S, Donn SM. Volume-controlled ventilation: variations on a theme. Clin Perinatol 2001;28:547–60.

[12] Keszler M, Abubakar K. Volume guarantee: Stability of tidal volume and incidence of hypocarbia. Pediatr Pulmonol 2004;38:240–5.

[13] Cheema IU, Ahluwalia JS. Feasibility of tidal volume-guided ventilation in newborn infants: a randomized, crossover trial using the volume guarantee modality. Pediatrics 2001;107:1323–8.

[14] Lista G, Colnaghi M, Castoldi F, et al. Impact of targeted-volume ventilation on lung inflammatory response in preterm infants with respiratory distress syndrome (RDS). Pediatr Pulmonol 2004;37:510–4.

[15] Herrera C, Gerhardt T, Claure N, et al. Effects of volume-guaranteed synchronized intermittent mandatory ventilation on preterm infants recovering from respiratory failure. Pediatrics 2002;110:529–33.

[16] Olsen SL, Thibeault DW, Truog WE. Crossover trial comparing pressure support with synchronized intermittent mandatory ventilation. J Perinatol 2002;22:461–6.

[17] McCallion N, Davis P, Morley C. Volume-targeted versus pressure-limited ventilation in the neonate. Cochrane Database Syst Rev 2005;CD003666.

[18] Sinha SK, Donn SM, Gavey J, et al. Randomised trial of volume controlled versus time cycled, pressure limited ventilation in preterm infants with respiratory distress syndrome. Arch Dis Child Fetal Neonatal Ed 1997;77:F202–5.

[19] Piotrowski A, Sobala W, Kawczynski P. Patient-initiated, pressure-regulated, volume-controlled ventilation compared with intermittent mandatory ventilation in neonates: a prospective, randomised study. Intensive Care Med 1997;23:975–81.

[20] Singh J, Sinha SK, Clarke P, et al. Mechanical ventilation of very low birth weight infants: is volume or pressure a better target variable? J Pediatr 2006;149:308–13.

[21] Weiswasser J, Lueders M, Stolar CJ. Pressure- versus volume-cycled ventilation in liquid-ventilated neonatal piglet lungs. J Pediatr Surg 1998;33:1158–62.

[22] Hummler HD, Engelmann A, Pohlandt F, et al. Volume-controlled intermittent mandatory ventilation in preterm infants with hypoxemic episodes. Intensive Care Med 2006;32:577–84.

[23] Davis PG, Morley C. Volume control: a logical solution to volutrauma. J Pediatr 2006;149: 290–1.

ELSEVIER
SAUNDERS

CLINICS IN
PERINATOLOGY

Clin Perinatol 34 (2007) 107–116

Volume Guarantee Ventilation

Martin Keszler, MD*, Kabir M. Abubakar, MD

*Division of Neonatal-Perinatal Medicine,
Georgetown University Hospital, Washington DC 20007, USA*

The advent of volume-targeted modalities of conventional ventilation that, for the first time, allow effective control of delivered tidal volume (V_T) when ventilating even extremely low birth weight infants, is one of the most exciting developments in neonatal respiratory support. Refinements of volume-controlled ventilation have made it possible to use this approach even in small preterm infants who previously could not be effectively ventilated in this way. A number of modifications of pressure-limited ventilation have been developed in recent years to combine the advantages of pressure-limited ventilation with the benefits of controlling delivered tidal volume. These modalities are designed to deliver a target tidal volume by microprocessor-directed adjustments of inspiratory pressure or time. Each of the available modalities has advantages and disadvantages. In this chapter, we will specifically focus on Volume Guarantee ventilation. We will outline the rationale for volume-targeted ventilation, provide a detailed description of ventilator function, summarize available clinical studies, and discuss the clinical application of Volume Guarantee. General aspects of volume-targeted ventilation and description of other modes of volume-targeted ventilation can be found in another article in this volume.

Rationale for volume-targeted ventilation

Time-cycled, pressure-limited, continuous flow ventilation became the standard neonatal ventilatory mode in the 1970s and 1980s. Early attempts to use traditional volume-controlled ventilation proved to be impractical in small preterm infants, as a result of loss of tidal volume to compression of gas in the circuit and the leak around uncuffed endotracheal tubes.

* Corresponding author. Georgetown University Hospital, Room M-3400, 3800 Reservoir Road, NW, Washington, DC 20007.

E-mail address: keszlerm@gunet.georgetown.edu (M. Keszler).

Pressure-limited ventilation has remained the standard method of newborn mechanical ventilation for more than 30 years, because of its relative simplicity, ability to ventilate effectively despite significant leaks around uncuffed endotracheal tubes, improved intrapulmonary gas distribution from the decelerating gas flow pattern, and the presumed benefit of directly controlling peak inspiratory pressure. In addition, the infant always has a source of fresh gas from which to breathe spontaneously between mechanical breaths. The major disadvantage of pressure-limited ventilation lies in the variable tidal volume that results from changes in lung compliance and resistance. Such changes may occur quite rapidly, especially in the immediate postnatal period as a result of clearing of lung fluid, optimization of lung volume, and administration of the exogenous surfactant preparations. The potential consequences of such rapid improvements in compliance include inadvertent hyperventilation and lung damage from excessively large tidal volumes (volutrauma). Even a half-dozen excessively large breaths have been shown to cause sustained adverse effects on lung function in premature lambs [1], suggesting that it may not be possible to respond rapidly enough with manual adjustment of inspiratory pressure to prevent lung damage. Hypocapnia also continues to be a common problem despite increasing awareness of its dangers; a recent study documented inadvertent hyperventilation to arterial partial pressure of carbon dioxide ($PaCO_2$) less than 25 mm Hg in 30% of ventilated newborn infants during the first day of life [2].

The ability to directly control inspiratory pressure has been considered for a long time to be an important benefit of pressure-limited ventilation. Despite extensive evidence that excessive volume, rather than pressure, is the key determinant of ventilator-induced lung injury (VILI), preoccupation with pressure as the main factor in VILI and air leak remains widespread. Dreyfuss and Saumon [3] demonstrated as early as 1988 that severe acute lung injury occurred in small animals ventilated with large tidal volumes, regardless of whether that volume was generated by positive or negative inspiratory pressure. On the other hand, animals whose chest wall and diaphragmatic excursion were limited by external binding to minimize large swings in tidal volume experienced much less acute lung damage when exposed to the same high inspiratory pressure. This landmark paper and other similar experiments clearly show that excessive tidal volume, not pressure by itself, is primarily responsible for lung injury [4,5]. However, it has been only recently that full appreciation of the importance of volutrauma and the dangers of inadvertent hyperventilation [6,7] have brought about renewed interest in directly controlling tidal volume.

Functional description of Volume Guarantee ventilation

The Volume Guarantee (VG) option available on the Draeger Babylog 8000-plus (Draeger Medical, Luebeck, Germany) may be combined with any of the standard ventilator modes (Assist/Control [A/C], Synchronized Intermittent Mandatory Ventilation [SIMV], and Pressure Support Ventilation [PSV]). The VG mode is a pressure-limited, volume-targeted, time- or flow-cycled form of ventilation. The operator chooses a target tidal volume and selects a pressure limit up to which the inspiratory pressure (the working pressure) may be adjusted. The microprocessor compares *exhaled* tidal volume of the previous breath to the desired target and adjusts the working pressure up or down to try to achieve the target tidal volume (Fig. 1). Exhaled tidal volume is used for autoregulation of inspiratory pressure, because it more closely approximates true tidal volume in the presence of significant leak around the endotracheal tube, a common problem in newborns with uncuffed endotracheal tubes [8]. The algorithm limits the pressure increment from one breath to the next to a maximum of 3 cm H_2O, to avoid overcorrection leading to excessive tidal volume and oscillations of the system (in engineering terms, this is referred to as dampening). This limit, and the fact that the exhaled tidal volume of the prior breath is used, means that with very rapid changes in compliance or patient inspiratory effort, several breaths may be needed to reach the target tidal volume after a sudden change. Breaths triggered by the infant (assisted breaths) and untriggered mechanical breaths are each controlled separately to minimize fluctuations in V_T. To minimize the risk of excessively large tidal volume, the microprocessor opens the expiratory valve, terminating any additional gas delivery if the *inspired* tidal volume exceeds 130% of the previous breath. The algorithm is designed to make slower incremental adjustment for low tidal volume and more rapid adjustment for excessive,

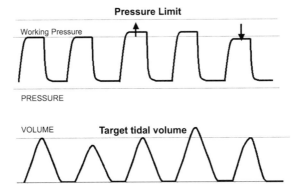

Fig. 1. Principles of operation of volume guarantee. The device automatically adjusts the inspiratory pressure, based on exhaled tidal volume of the previous breath, to deliver the tidal volume that is set by the user. As illustrated, the V_T of the first breath is on target, thus no adjustment is made. The second breath falls short of the target V_T, leading to an increase in working pressure of the next breath. The third breath is on target, thus there is no change in working pressure. The fourth breath is above the target, leading to a drop in the working pressure for the fifth breath, bringing the V_T back to the target value. (*Modified from* Keszler M. Volume targeted ventilation. Early Hum Dev 2006;82:811–8; with permission.)

potentially dangerous V_T. The term "guarantee" is somewhat misleading, because the V_T fluctuates around the target value in spontaneously breathing infants with a variable respiratory drive. Nonetheless, the V_T has been documented to be much less variable with, than without VG [9]. Autoregulation of inspiratory pressure makes VG a self-weaning modality. Because weaning occurs in real-time, rather than intermittently in response to blood gases or intermittent observation of delivered tidal volume, the VG modality may achieve faster weaning from mechanical ventilation. Although more tolerant of endotracheal tube leak than some volume-targeted devices because of the use of exhaled V_T measurement, VG becomes impractical in the presence of a leak that substantially exceeds 40%, because in this situation the V_T measurement increasingly underestimates the actual delivered V_T. A leak of that magnitude that cannot be corrected by repositioning the infant or the endotracheal tube indicates that the endotracheal tube is too small. The problem can usually be corrected by re-intubating the infant with a larger endotracheal tube.

It must be emphasized that the interaction between all ventilators and a spontaneously breathing infant are complex and not easily studied. Although a very stable V_T can be achieved in a paralyzed patient with a snugly fitting endotracheal tube even in the face of rather rapid changes in compliance or airway resistance, this is not the usual situation in the newborn intensive care unit. With synchronized ventilation, the V_T that enters the infant's lungs is the combined result of the negative inspiratory effort of the infant and the positive pressure generated by the ventilator. Because the preterm infant's contribution to this transpulmonary pressure is highly variable and inconsistent, the V_T of a spontaneously breathing ventilated infant is extremely variable. Especially during the recovery phase of lung disease, even small preterm infants, particularly when agitated, are capable of spontaneously generating large tidal volumes that may briefly exceed 20 mL/kg. Some extremely premature, ventilator-dependent infants develop frequent episodes of forced exhalation, or a sort of Valsalva maneuver [10]. The reason for this behavior is unclear, but it results in near-complete cessation of gas flow for the duration of the episode and is commonly accompanied by falling oxygen saturation and bradycardia. Because the forceful exhalation results in substantial loss of lung volume and compliance, recovery usually takes several minutes. Similar loss of functional residual capacity occurs with endotracheal tube suctioning. Our group recently demonstrated faster recovery from these forced exhalation episodes and from suctioning of the endotracheal tube with VG, compared with standard pressure-limited ventilation [11,12]. Although clearly helpful in reducing the impact of these perturbations, VG could not eliminate substantial fluctuations in delivered V_T. McCallion and colleagues [13] identified an additional source of fluctuation in tidal volume targeting by VG. They observed that in 3% of breaths, expiration was briefly interrupted by what was presumed to be diaphragmatic "braking" by the infant, causing the microprocessor to misidentify this interrupted exhalation as a full breath and to use only a part of the actual tidal volume to regulate the pressure for the next breath (although the 3-cm H_2O incremental limit will prevent major overshoot). It is therefore important to understand the complexity of patient-ventilator interactions and recognize that even with volume-targeted ventilation, considerable variability of individual tidal volumes is to be expected in the awake, spontaneously breathing infant.

Clinical studies of VG ventilation

All studies of volume-targeted ventilation to date have focused on feasibility and short-term outcomes, rather than major long-term benefits. In a 4-hour crossover trial, Cheema and Ahluwalia [14] compared A/C with and without VG in a group of infants with acute respiratory distress syndrome (RDS), and separately evaluated SIMV with and without VG during the weaning phase in 40 premature newborn infants. During both VG periods, the infants achieved equivalent gas exchange using slightly lower peak airway pressure and with fewer excessively large tidal volumes. The authors concluded the VG modality was feasible and may offer the benefit of lower airway pressures. No major conclusions could be drawn from this short-term study, other than that the ventilator performs as intended and no short-term adverse effects were evident.

Herrera and colleagues [15] compared the effects of SIMV+VG with SIMV alone on ventilation and gas exchange in a group of very low birth weight infants recovering from acute respiratory failure. Short-term use of SIMV+VG resulted in automatic reduction of the mechanical support and enhancement of spontaneous respiratory effort, while maintaining gas exchange relatively unchanged in comparison to SIMV alone. Further shift of the work of breathing to the patient was documented when the target V_T was reduced from the normal 4.5 mL/kg target to 3 mL/kg. The proportion of excessively large breaths greater than 7 mL/kg was significantly lower with SIMV+VG, compared with SIMV alone (6% versus 16%). The study added further confirmation of the feasibility, potential, and short-term benefits of VG, but again, only short-term physiologic outcomes were studied.

In a small prospective clinical trial involving 34 fairly large preterm infants (mean birth weight 1122 g), Nafday and colleagues [16] compared SIMV to PSV+VG over the first 24 hours of life. They did not demonstrate a difference in the primary outcome, the time to extubation, or other important clinical outcomes, but this "pilot" study lacked adequate statistical power. Furthermore, the original group assignment was only maintained for the first 24 hours, likely negating any possible differences. The authors noted that mean airway pressure declined more rapidly in the SIMV group, but this was simply the result of lowering the ventilator rate (leading to lower I:E ratio) with SIMV. There was no difference in the rate of decline of peak pressure. Significantly fewer blood gases were needed in the VG group.

Olsen and colleagues [17] compared 4-hour periods of PSV+VG with SIMV alone in a crossover trial of 14 infants with a mean gestational age of 34 weeks. The arterial/alveolar oxygen difference, arterial carbon dioxide tension, and specific dynamic compliance were similar during both periods. Minute ventilation and mean airway pressure were higher and end-expiratory volume was lower during PSV+VG compared with SIMV. The authors concluded that use of PSV+VG could not be routinely recommended. The findings of this study should be viewed with caution because of significant concerns about the study design, data acquisition, and interpretation [18]. Ventilator variables were periodically manually recorded from values displayed by the ventilator and then averaged, instead of being continuously electronically imported. During VG, the working pressure and V_T vary from breath to breath in spontaneously breathing infants; recording these manually can produce significant error. The reportedly lower V_T during SIMV resulted from inclusion of both spontaneous and mechanical breaths. At the same time, the calculated minute ventilation was underestimated for SIMV because only the set IMV rate was used for calculation. Because of the low levels of PEEP used in this study, some loss of lung volume was likely as a result of shorter inspiratory time in PSV and the lower peak inspiratory pressure (PIP) used in VG. This effect could have been mitigated by using a more appropriate level of positive end-expiratory pressure (PEEP) to maintain lung volume.

Our group earlier showed that VG combined with A/C, SIMV, or PSV in a short-term crossover study led to significantly less variability of tidal volume with VG, compared with A/C or SIMV alone and that peak inspiratory pressures were similar [9]. In a subsequent small clinical trial, we explored the hypothesis that VG combined with A/C would maintain V_T and $PaCO_2$ within a narrow target range more consistently than A/C alone during the first 72 hours of life in preterm infants with uncomplicated RDS [19]. This first prospective randomized trial of VG demonstrated that excessively large tidal volume and hypocapnia could be significantly reduced, although not entirely eliminated, with the use of VG (Fig. 2). These findings support the potential of VG to reduce many of the important adverse effects of mechanical ventilation, but again involve only short-term outcomes.

Next, in a short-term crossover trial we studied 12 extremely low birth weight (ELBW) infants with a mean birth weight of 679 ± 138 g to determine whether VG is more effective when combined with A/C or SIMV [20]. As anticipated, V_T was more stable when VG was combined with A/C, because the interval between supported breaths is longer during SIMV, leading to slower adjustment. An unexpected finding was that during SIMV, the infants had lower and more variable oxygen saturation and had significantly more tachycardia and tachypnea. By design, the V_T was identical, but significantly higher PIP was required during SIMV to achieve the same V_T. The tachypnea, tachycardia, and lower, more variable oxygen saturation suggest

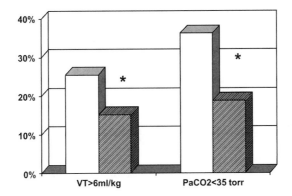

Fig. 2. Volume Guarantee (solid bars) resulted in significant reduction of breaths with tidal volume above 6 mL/kg and $PaCO_2$ values less than 35 mm Hg, when compared with A/C alone (clear bars). *$P < .001$.

that the reason for the higher machine PIP was that the infants were tiring during the SIMV period and contributing less effort by the end of the 2-hour period when the measurements were obtained. This conclusion is based on the realization that during synchronized ventilation, the delivered V_T is the result of the combined inspiratory effort of the baby and the positive ventilator pressure; as the baby tires and contributes less, the ventilator needs to generate higher PIP to deliver the same V_T.

To address the concern regarding possible untoward effects of the additional instrumental dead-space (IDS) of the flow sensor and to establish normative data for target V_T in ELBW infants, we reviewed 451 paired observations of V_T and arterial blood gas measurements in 47 infants weighing less than 800 g at birth (mean weight 627 g, range 400–790 g) during the fist 24 hours of life [21]. The V_T/kg needed to maintain normocapnia was inversely related to weight ($r = -0.56$, $P < .01$), indicating some effect of the fixed IDS. Mean V_T of infants weighing 500 g or less was 5.7 ± 0.36 mL/kg compared with 4.7 ± 0.39 mL/kg for those weighing 700 g or more ($P < .001$). The absolute mean set and measured V_T was 3.12 ± 0.76 mL and 3.13 ± 0.66 mL, respectively, barely above the estimated instrumental plus anatomical dead space of 3.01 mL. While maintaining normocapnia, 48% of all tidal volumes were below the estimated dead space. We concluded that there is a greater impact of IDS in the tiniest infants, but there is no need to forgo synchronized and volume-targeted ventilation because of concerns about the added dead space of the flow sensor. Effective alveolar ventilation occurs with V_T at or below dead space, suggesting that a spike of fresh gas penetrates through the dead space gas, similar to what occurs with high-frequency ventilation.

Cheema and colleagues [22] examined the effect of VG on the incidence of hypocapnia on the first arterial blood gas after initiation of mechanical ventilation. The incidence of hypocapnia was 32% with A/C+VG, compared with 57% with A/C alone, but this difference fell short of statistical significance in this very small prospective trial. Cheema and colleagues noted a significant negative correlation between gestational age and $PaCO_2$, although they did not appear to appreciate the reason for this observation. The fact that the most premature and smallest infants had higher $PaCO_2$ values undoubtedly reflects the impact of the fixed instrumental dead space documented in the above-mentioned study [21].

Dawson and Davies [23] also examined the relationship between tidal volume, minute ventilation, and $PaCO_2$ in patients ventilated with VG. They reported that 96.5% of the blood gases during the first 48 hours were within their acceptable range of 25 to 65 mm Hg when the V_T was set at a mean value of 4 mL/kg. More importantly, only 1 (0.3%) of 288 $PaCO_2$ values were less than 25 mm Hg. Unfortunately, because the VG was combined with SIMV and the data were collected retrospectively from set IMV rates and tidal volumes, very little correlation was noted between calculated minute ventilation and $PaCO_2$. No adjustment was made for the effect of fixed instrumental dead space for ELBW infants, which may explain why the correlation between set V_T and $PaCO_2$ was also poor.

Recently, we explored the evolution of V_T requirement over time, evaluating a total of 1033 paired blood gas and V_T observations in 30 ELBW infants (mean birth weight 736 ± 110 g) over the first 3 weeks of life [24]. The mean V_T rose from 5.01 mL/kg during the first 24 hours to 5.73 mL/kg during the third week of life, while mean $PaCO_2$ rose from 43.4 to 53.9 mm Hg. Thus, despite permissive hypercapnia, progressively higher V_T was needed, likely because of a combination of progressive dilation of the upper airways (increased anatomical deadspace) and increased alveolar dead space as a consequence of heterogeneous aeration of the lungs with evolving chronic lung disease.

Lista and colleagues [25] recently provided a convincing study about the potential benefits of volume-targeted ventilation. They randomly assigned 53 preterm infants with RDS to PSV alone or PSV combined with VG, using set tidal volume of 5 mL/kg. They reported decreased levels of pro-inflammatory cytokines in the tracheal aspirate of infants in the VG group. The duration of mechanical ventilation was 12.3 ± 3.0 days in the PSV-only group compared with 8.8 ± 3.0 days in those on PSV plus VG. In the authors' original analysis, this fell short of statistical significance, but subsequent reanalysis by Cochrane Systematic Reviews demonstrated that this was a significant reduction in the duration of mechanical ventilation [26]. These data strongly support the hypothesis that VG may reduce ventilator-induced lung injury, which is mediated by the release of pro-inflammatory cytokines in a process known as biotrauma [5].

Interestingly, a subsequent similar study by the same authors now using a target tidal volume of 3 mL/kg showed an *increase* in pro-inflammatory cytokines [27], most likely as a consequence of atelectasis that resulted from the combination of low V_T and a low end-expiratory pressure of 3 to 4 cm H_2O that was used [28].

Summary

VG is one of several forms of volume-targeted ventilation shown to be feasible and safe even in ELBW infants, who now represent the majority of ventilated infants in our neonatal intensive care units and who are at greatest risk of developing chronic lung disease. VG ventilation has been demonstrated to function as intended and to lead to shorter duration of mechanical ventilation and more stable tidal volume delivery with a lower incidence of hypocarbia and excessively large tidal volumes. When combined with other lung-protective strategies aimed at optimizing lung volume and ensuring even distribution of the delivered tidal volume, volume-targeted ventilation appears to offer hope of making a substantial impact on ventilator-induced lung injury. Nevertheless, definitive evidence of major, long-term clinical benefit(s) of VG is not available at this time. It must be emphasized that the development of chronic lung disease in extremely preterm infants is multifactorial. The degree of prematurity and consequences of intrauterine inflammation have very large effects, potentially dwarfing any impact of ventilation strategy. Consequently, multicenter studies involving a large number of infants will be needed to have sufficient statistical power to detect modest, but clinically important differences in the incidence of chronic lung disease. Surrogate outcomes, such as more rapid weaning from mechanical ventilation, may be the closest we can come to validating the benefits of volume-targeted ventilation.

Also see online addendum "Clinical Guidelines for the Use of Volume Guarantee: Practice Guidelines for the Bedside" at www.perinatology. theclinics.com.

References

[1] Bjorklund LJ, Ingimarsson J, Curstedt T, et al. Manual ventilation with a few large breaths at birth compromises the therapeutic effect of subsequent surfactant replacement in immature lambs. Pediatr Res 1997;42:348–55.

[2] Luyt K, Wright D, Baumer JH. Randomised study comparing extent of hypocarbia in preterm infants during conventional and patient triggered ventilation. Arch Dis Child Fetal Neonatal Ed 2001;84:F14–7.

[3] Dreyfuss D, Saumon G. Ventilator-induced lung injury: lessons from experimental studies. Am J Respir Crit Care Med 1998;157:294–323.

[4] Clark RH, Slutsky AS, Gertsmann DR. Lung protective strategies of ventilation in the neonate: what are they? Pediatrics 2000;105:112–4.

[5] Slutsky AS. Ventilator-induced lung injury: from barotrauma to biotrauma. Respir Care 2005;50:646–59.

[6] Graziani LJ, Spitzer AR, Mitchell DG, et al. Mechanical ventilation in preterm infants. Neurosonographic and developmental studies. Pediatrics 1992;90:515–22.

[7] Wiswell TE, Graziani LJ, Kornhauser MS, et al. Effects of hypocarbia on the development of cystic periventricular leukomalacia in premature infants treated with high-frequency jet ventilation. Pediatrics 1996;98:918–24.

[8] Bernstein G, Knodel E, Heldt GP. Airway leak size in neonates and autocycling of three flow-triggered ventilators. Crit Care Med 1995;23:1739–44.

[9] Abubakar KM, Keszler M. Patient-ventilator interactions in new modes of patient-triggered ventilation. Pediatr Pulmonol 2001;32(1):71–5.

[10] Dimaguila MA, DiFiore JA, Martin R, et al. Characteristics of hypoxemic episodes in very low birth weight infants on ventilatory support. J Pediatr 1997;130:577–83.

[11] Keszler M, Abubakar KM. Volume guarantee accelerates recovery from forced exhalation episodes. Pediatr Res 2004;55:545A.

[12] Abubakar K, Montazami S, Keszler M. Volume guarantee accelerates recovery from endotracheal tube suctioning in ventilated preterm infants. E-PAS 2006;59:5560.343.

[13] McCallion N, Lau R, Dargaville PA, et al. Volume guarantee ventilation, interrupted expiration and expiratory braking. Arch Dis Child 2005;90(8):865–70.

[14] Cheema IU, Ahluwalia JS. Feasibility of tidal volume-guided ventilation in newborn infants: a randomized, crossover trial using the volume guarantee modality. Pediatrics 2001;107: 1323–8.

[15] Herrera CM, Gerhardt T, Claure N, et al. Effects of volume-guaranteed synchronized intermittent mandatory ventilation in preterm infants recovering from respiratory failure. Pediatrics 2002;110:529–33.

[16] Nafday SM, Green RS, Lin J, et al. Is there an advantage of using pressure support ventilation with volume guarantee in the initial management of premature infants with respiratory distress syndrome? A pilot study. J Perinatol 2005;25:193–7.

[17] Olsen SL, Thibeault DW, Truog WE. Crossover trial comparing pressure support with synchronized intermittent mandatory ventilation. J Perinatol 2002;22(6):461–6.

[18] Keszler M, Abubakar KM, Mammel MC. Response to Olsen, et al. Study comparing SIMV & PSV. J Perinatol 2003;23:434–5.

[19] Keszler M, Abubakar KM. Volume guarantee: stability of tidal volume and incidence of hypocarbia. Pediatr Pulmonol 2004;38:240–5.

[20] Abubakar K, Keszler M. Effect of volume guarantee combined with assist/control vs. synchronized intermittent mandatory ventilation. J Perinatol 2005;25:638–42.

[21] Montazami S, Abubakar K, Keszler M. Impact of instrumental dead space on volume guarantee mode of ventilation in extremely low birth weight infants. E-PAS 2006;59:468.

[22] Cheema IU, Sinha AK, Kempley ST, et al. Impact of volume guarantee ventilation on arterial carbon dioxide tension in newborn infants: a randomized controlled trial. Early Hum Dev, in press.

[23] Dawson C, Davies MW. Volume-targeted ventilation and arterial carbon dioxide in neonates. J Paediatr Child Health 2005;41(9–10):518–21.

[24] Montazami S, Abubakar K, Keszler M. Changes in tidal volume requirement with advancing postnatal age in ventilated extremely low birth weight (ELBW) infants. E-PAS 2006;59: 5560.339.

[25] Lista G, Colnaghi M, Castoldi F, et al. Impact of targeted-volume ventilation on lung inflammatory response in preterm infants with respiratory distress syndrome. Pediatr Pulmonol 2004;37:510–4.

[26] McCallion N, Davis PG, Morley CJ. Volume-targeted versus pressure-limited ventilation in the neonate. Cochrane Database Syst Rev 2005;CD003666.

[27] Lista G, Castoldi F, Fontana P, et al. Lung inflammation in preterm infants with respiratory distress syndrome: effects of ventilation with different tidal volumes. Pediatr Pulmonol 2006; 41:357–63.

[28] Keszler M. Volume guarantee and ventilator-induced lung injury: Goldilocks' rules apply [commentary]. Pediatr Pulmonol 2006;41:364–6.

CLINICS IN
PERINATOLOGY

Clin Perinatol 34 (2007) 117–128

In Support of Pressure Support

Subrata Sarkar, MD, Steven M. Donn, MD*

*Department of Pediatrics, Division of Neonatal-Perinatal Medicine, F5790 C.S. Mott
Children's Hospital, University of Michigan Health System, 1500 East Medical Center Drive,
Ann Arbor, MI 48109-0254, USA*

For many decades clinicians struggled with the best way to support spontaneous breathing during mechanical ventilation. The advent of continuous bias flow was a step forward, providing a source of fresh gas from which the patient could breathe between mechanical breaths, and these spontaneous breaths could be supported with positive end-expiratory pressure (PEEP) to maintain some degree of alveolar expansion and decrease the work of breathing.

In the newborn infant, the institution of mechanical ventilation comes with a cost. The narrow-lumen, high-resistance endotracheal tube can contribute to an increased work of breathing. The ventilator circuit and its attachments often add dead space, and work may be involved in opening a demand valve in demand-flow systems or in reaching the assist sensitivity in patient-triggered systems. Collectively, these elements comprise the imposed work of breathing.

In 1989, Kacmarek and colleagues [1] described pressure support ventilation (PSV) for the management of adult patients who required mechanical ventilation. PSV was designed to provide an inspiratory pressure assist during spontaneous breathing to overcome the imposed work of breathing. Refinements in ventilator technology and signal detection enabled the use of PSV in the neonatal population in the early 1990s.

Characteristics of pressure support ventilation

PSV is delivered to the mechanically ventilated patient during spontaneous breathing. It is a triggered mode, with changes in airway pressure or flow used as the trigger signal. Following detection of spontaneous patient effort, the ventilator delivers a breath that is flow cycled but time limited.

---

* Corresponding author.
E-mail address: smdonnmd@med.umich.edu (S.M. Donn).

As shown in Fig. 1, there is a sharp increase in inspiratory flow, which peaks and then decelerates rapidly. At the termination point, inspiratory flow ceases, and the breath cycles directly into expiration. The specific termination point is determined by the algorithm within the ventilator, and it is usually a function of the delivered tidal volume. For virtually all neonatal patients, this occurs when inspiratory flow has decelerated to 5% of peak flow (or when there has been a 95% decay in the decelerating portion of the inspiratory flow waveform). The clinician may limit the inspiratory time, and if so, the limit variable will be whichever condition occurs first. Inspiratory flow delivery during PSV is variable and is proportional to the patient's effort and pulmonary mechanics.

The clinician chooses the amount of pressure that is delivered during PSV. If the pressure is chosen to deliver a full tidal volume breath, it is referred to as PS_{max} (Fig. 2A). If the pressure is chosen solely to overcome the imposed work of breathing, it is referred to as PS_{min}. Levels in between provide partial respiratory support of spontaneous breathing (Fig. 2B).

PSV is thus a spontaneous ventilatory mode in which an inspiratory pressure boost is provided to overcome the imposed work of breathing or to provide additional support to a mechanically ventilated patient. The patient has control over the rate, because it is patient triggered, and the inspiratory time, because it is flow cycled. The clinician has control over the inspiratory pressure and time limit and the synchronized intermittent mandatory ventilation (SIMV) rate.

PSV is generally used in conjunction with SIMV, usually as a weaning strategy. SIMV is used to provide a backup or safety net in the event of patient apnea or decreased effort. In patients who have intact and reliable respiratory drive, PSV may be used alone.

Several different approaches have been used to wean adult patients from mechanical ventilation using PSV. One approach is to continue SIMV while

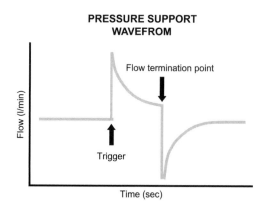

Fig. 1. Pressure support flow waveform. Note the sharply rising accelerating inspiratory flow and the termination point, which ends inspiratory flow and cycles directly into expiration.

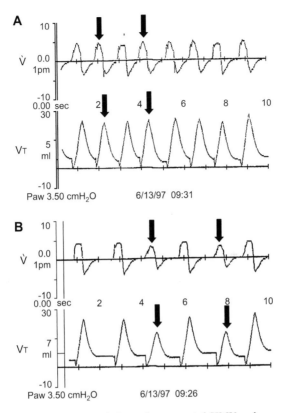

Fig. 2. Flow and volume waveforms during volume-targeted SIMV and pressure support ventilation. (A) PS$_{max}$. Note that tidal volume delivery is the same during the SIMV breaths (*arrows*) and the PSV-supported spontaneous breaths. (B) Partial pressure support. Note that the delivered tidal volumes in PSV (*arrows*) are less than the SIMV breaths.

weaning the pressure level in PSV. Another has been to maintain PS$_{max}$ while maintaining a moderate SIMV rate, which is then weaned to allow the patient to assume a greater proportion of breathing, followed by reduction in PSV pressure until PS$_{min}$ is reached.

Pressure support ventilation: adult and pediatric experience

A commonly used ventilation modality in adults and children is volume-controlled ventilation. Addition of PSV, which is a switch to a pressure-targeted modality, has been shown to decrease the spontaneous work of breathing by partial or total unloading of respiratory muscles in adults and children.

Total unloading correlated well with levels of inspiratory assist, and when PSV was used at levels sufficient enough for total unloading of respiratory muscles it led to a muscle-resting effect similar to volume-controlled ventilation [2,3].

Tokiaka and colleagues [4] in 1989 compared the effects of PSV with those of assist/control ventilation (A/C) in eight adults who had acute respiratory failure. They noted that with a pressure support level that was comparable with the peak pressure of volume-assisted breaths, tidal volume was significantly higher, respiratory frequency was lower, and patient–ventilator synchrony improved significantly during PSV. Improvement in patient–ventilator synchrony, perceived improvement in patient comfort, better quality of sleep, reduced need for sedation, and the simplicity of PSV have led to its wide acceptance by the adult medical community [3,5]. High-level pressure support also provides ventilation/perfusion ratio distribution similar to SIMV and leads to adequate oxygenation and ventilation [6].

PSV has been used in patients who have status asthmaticus and also in post–cardiac surgery patients. In asthmatic patients, PSV improved hypercapnia at significantly lower airway pressure compared with A/C ventilation [7]. PSV was also well tolerated and did not cause hemodynamic compromise in post–cardiac surgical patients [8].

Because of the plausible advantage of combining PSV with other modes of synchronized ventilation during the weaning phase of ventilatory support, many studies comparing PSV with other weaning modes have been performed in adults and children. In a large multicenter prospective randomized controlled trial (RCT), PSV was compared with daily spontaneous breathing trials through a T-piece and with SIMV in 109 difficult-to-wean adults during the weaning phase of mechanical ventilation [9]. In this trial, PSV was associated with a significantly lower number of weaning failures, shorter weaning duration, and a shorter total length of intensive care unit stay compared with other modes. In contrast, two other large prospective RCTs did not find PSV to be superior in adults [10,11]. Differences between the seemingly conflicting results of these trials stem from the use of different weaning protocols in each study and the dissimilarity between comparative patient groups. In children, PSV and volume support ventilation (VSV) are the most commonly used modes to wean from mechanical ventilation. Studies have shown that gradual weaning from mechanical ventilation may not be indicated in most young infants and children who have acute respiratory failure [12]. In contrast to adult patients, in the largest RCT performed to date in infants and children most children could be weaned from mechanical ventilator support in 2 days or less, and the weaning protocols (PSV protocol, VSV protocol, or no protocol) did not significantly shorten this brief duration of weaning [12].

The rationale for the use of PSV and its benefits are well documented in adults, especially during weaning from mechanical ventilatory support. Extrapolation of ventilatory modes and weaning methods commonly used in adults and preterm infants, including PSV, may not be appropriate in young infants and children because of their unique respiratory physiology, pulmonary mechanics, and epidemiology of acute lung disease [12].

Pressure support ventilation: neonatal experience

Perhaps because of the relative novelty of PSV, little information has been published regarding its use in newborns. PSV has been used independently as a stand-alone mode in newborn infants and can be used in conjunction with other modalities of pressure-limited or volume-controlled synchronized ventilation.

Pressure support ventilation as a stand-alone mode

PSV is a flow-cycled but time-limited mode that supports each spontaneous breath just like A/C, and may be used in newborn infants as a stand-alone technique when reliable respiratory drive is present. Pressure support ventilation is patient-triggered, in that the inspiratory time, respiratory rate, and, to some extent, the minute ventilation remain under the control of the patient, thereby facilitating a natural pattern of breathing.

Patient-triggered ventilation has been shown to result in a lower clinical distress score and better stress response with lower stress hormone concentrations in preterm babies [13]. PSV differs from time-cycled, pressure-targeted modes. In contrast to time cycling, flow cycling eliminates the gap between the end of inspiratory flow and the start of expiratory flow. This results in a more natural breathing pattern, and because the patient controls the inspiratory time during spontaneous breathing, patient comfort and patient–ventilator synchrony are enhanced during PSV. Typically, the pressure support level has been set at 30% to 50% of the difference between peak inspiratory pressure (PIP) and PEEP [14], or at a level to deliver an adequate tidal volume. As with A/C, weaning can be accomplished with gradual reduction of the pressure support level and allowing the infant to assume more of the work of breathing. Infants who have chronic lung disease may be particularly responsive to PSV because it provides the higher inspiratory flow rates that these patients usually need, resulting in decreased work of breathing and improved lung mechanics. In a case report of a preterm infant who had bronchopulmonary dysplasia (BPD), switching the mode of ventilation from volume-controlled SIMV to PSV alone resulted in significant improvement in the delivered tidal volume at a lower PIP and improved compliance, which facilitated prompt weaning and extubation [15]. PSV was also shown to augment spontaneous breathing with improved thoracoabdominal synchrony in nine term infants who had undergone cardiac surgery but were awake with stable hemodynamic and respiratory parameters and ready for weaning from the ventilator. Three successive levels of PSV (0, 5, and 10 cm H_2O) were randomly applied over a 30-minute period. The tidal volume (V_T) increased by 23% with PSV of 5 cm H_2O and by

69% at 10 cm H_2O, associated with an increase in minute ventilation compared with no PSV [16]. The thoracic cage in neonates is more compliant than in older children. In addition, a higher inspiratory load from increased airway resistance results in thoracoabdominal asynchrony. Thoracoabdominal asynchrony has the potential to lead to inefficient diaphragmatic motion and results in respiratory muscle fatigue easily in premature infants [17]. All of these problems can be ameliorated with use of PSV as demonstrated in this study.

PSV as a stand-alone mode may result in hypoventilation, particularly in sick extremely low birth weight (ELBW) infants who have insufficient and unreliable respiratory drive or effort for adequate triggering of the ventilator. In these infants, a backup ventilator rate (generally SIMV) is usually provided. Jurban and colleagues [18] demonstrated that too low a termination criterion can lead to increased expiratory effort with recruitment of accessory muscles of expiration. Too high a termination criterion may result in premature breath termination with increased ventilatory drive. This phenomenon has been best illustrated by Kapasi and colleagues [19] in a study of seven clinically stable neonates (31.4 ± 2 weeks gestation, weighing 1.49 ± 0.38 kg) in whom patient–ventilator synchrony, work of breathing, and patient effort were compared during different forms of patient-triggered ventilation in a random order for 20 minutes. Patient effort and work of breathing differed significantly among modes of ventilation [19]. PSV alone resulted in better patient–ventilator synchrony and lower inspiratory pressure time product and work of breathing (0.60 ± 0.39 cm $H_2O \cdot sec$, and 0.17 ± 0.14 J/L) compared to SIMV and IMV, but the effort and work of breathing were least with A/C (0.54 ± 0.29 cm $H_2O \cdot sec$, and 0.07 ± 0.04 J/L. A reduction in peak flow of 25% was required for inspiration to be terminated in this study, which resulted in inadequate inspiratory time, increased minute volume, and increased work of breathing during PSV compared to A/C. The results demonstrate the need to assess the patient's spontaneous inspiratory time and carefully set the end-inspiratory flow criteria to allow inspiratory time with PSV to coincide with the patient's desired inspiratory time [19]. It is also essential to assure that expiration is passive as evidenced by absence of a spike in end-expiratory pressure. Fortunately, most current ventilators offering PSV have incorporated the proper termination point into the pressure support algorithm as a function of the delivered tidal volume, eliminating the guesswork.

Another potential problem with PSV is auto-cycling, which results in automatic triggering. The presence of a gas leak, such as leaks around the endotracheal tube or ventilator circuit, flow oscillations from excessive vapor condensation in the ventilator circuit, or endogenous leaks (such as a bronchopleural fistula) may be misinterpreted by the ventilator as patient effort, resulting in the inadvertent delivery of positive pressure [20].

In summary, PSV represents a promising mode of ventilation that can be used as a stand-alone mode in stable and robust newborns, although its singular use is not advisable in critically ill preterm infants who have unreliable respiratory drive.

Pressure support ventilation during weaning

Successful weaning of the SIMV rate in preterm infants must be accompanied by an increase in spontaneous inspiratory effort to compensate for the reduction in mechanical support. Increased mechanical loads and poor spontaneous respiratory effort are common in preterm infants, however, and may delay the weaning process. The addition of PSV during weaning provides elastic unloading, averts diaphragmatic overexertion and fatigue, and facilitates the weaning process by alleviating some of the resistive work of breathing [21]. In a small study of 15 ELBW infants (birth weight 793 ± 217 g, gestational age 26.4 ± 1.5 weeks, postnatal age 15 ± 16 days), Osorio and colleagues [21] evaluated the short-term effects of two levels of PSV (3 and 6 cm H_2O) as an adjunct to SIMV on gas exchange and breathing effort during an acute reduction in the SIMV rate. Pressure support assistance of the spontaneous breathing effort over four consecutive 30-minute periods during an average 50% reduction in the SIMV rate helped to maintain adequate oxygenation and ventilation without a significant increase in inspiratory effort. PSV at 6 cm H_2O provided 93% elastic unloading with the average V_T of 4.3 mL/kg, whereas PSV at 3 cm H_2O provided 59% elastic unloading with a V_T of 3.6 mL/Kg. Partial mechanical unloading by PSV reduced the spontaneous per-breath effort. This reduction may be particularly important in infants in the acute phase of lung disease who have dynamically changing and impaired lung mechanics or a weak respiratory drive.

In another recent randomized crossover trial of PSV, breath-to-breath pulmonary mechanics data were collected from 10 premature infants during three modes of ventilation: SIMV alone, SIMV with partial PSV, and SIMV with full PSV (S. Gupta, S.K. Sinha, S.M. Donn, 2007, personal communication). Full PSV provided 5 to 8 mL/kg and partial PSV 2.5 to 4 mL/kg of expired tidal volume. In this study, a total of 19,112 breaths were analyzed. The minute ventilation increased and the spontaneous respiratory rate decreased as PSV was added and increased. The authors noted that PSV improved the efficiency of breathing during mechanical ventilation and the improvement was proportional to the level of PSV provided. Although these are small studies, they do support the use of combined modality to facilitate weaning from mechanical ventilation and demonstrate the relationship of differing levels of PSV.

Sinha and colleagues [22] in another RCT compared volume-targeted ventilation to time-cycled pressure-limited (TCPL) ventilation in 50 preterm infants weighing 1200 g or more who had clinical and radiographic evidence of RDS. PSV (minimum 10–12 cm H_2O above baseline) was used in the weaning phase, and the tidal volume delivery in each group was controlled at 5 to 8 mL/kg so that the only differences between the two groups were the ventilator modality and the manner in which the tidal volume was delivered. The two modes of ventilation were compared by determining the time required to achieve predetermined success criteria defined as alveolar–arterial oxygen difference less than 13 kPa for more than 12 hours, or mean $\overline{Paw}$ (airway pressure) less than 8 cm H_2O for more than 12 hours, or extubation for more than 12 hours. Infants weaned using PSV met the success criteria sooner. Use of PSV during the weaning phase might have contributed to the faster weaning, with an approximate 50% reduction in ventilation hours (mean time of 65.6 versus 125.6 hours, $P < .001$) in the volume-controlled group compared with TCPL group.

PSV as a supplement to other synchronized ventilation modalities to facilitate weaning from ventilatory support has gained widespread popularity. To date, the evidence base is small, yet supportive. More well-executed RCTs of PSV with adequate sample sizes and statistical power are warranted.

Pressure support ventilation as an adjunct to synchronized intermittent mandatory ventilation

The high airway resistance of narrow endotracheal tubes and the added load imposed by triggering devices, combined with inconsistent spontaneous respiratory effort and mechanical disadvantages conferred by poor chest wall stability are common in preterm infants and can lead to small, ineffective spontaneous tidal volumes. The spontaneous breath tidal volumes may not be sufficiently large to maintain adequate alveolar ventilation and may represent just dead space ventilation [23]. The addition of PSV to SIMV to augment spontaneous breaths effectively takes care of the problem of the added mechanical load, results in improvement in spontaneous breath tidal volumes, and avoids the need for larger SIMV tidal volumes. In a small anecdotal series, 10 infants (gestational age of 24 to 34 weeks and birth weight of 600 to 2000 g) who had BPD unresponsive to A/C ventilation and other medical interventions were switched to volume-controlled SIMV at rates and tidal volumes comparable to what they had been receiving earlier. PSV was then added in an attempt to deliver tidal volumes ranging from 5 to 8 mL/kg body weight and was subsequently reduced to a minimum of 8 cm H_2O according to infant's blood gas response and clinical condition. All 10 infants responded to the institution of PSV and were able to be successfully extubated after a median of 6 days (range 3–11) [24].

In a recent large RCT by Reyes and colleagues [25], 107 preterm ELBW infants who required mechanical ventilation for respiratory failure during the first postnatal week were assigned to SIMV or SIMV plus pressure support. Fifty-three infants were assigned to receive SIMV and 54 infants received SIMV plus PSV (birth weight 722 ± 125 g versus 749 ± 134 g, and gestational age 25 ± 1.4 versus 25.4 ± 1.3 weeks). Addition of pressure support led to earlier extubation during the first 28 days, but total duration of mechanical ventilation, duration of oxygen dependency, and oxygen need at 36 weeks' postmenstrual age alone or combined with death did not differ between the groups. The infants from the SIMV plus PSV group reached minimal ventilator settings earlier, however, and among the 700 to 1000 g birth weight stratum, oxygen dependency was also shorter. A specific ventilator management protocol was followed in this study until the 28th postnatal day, and the clinical team determined the subsequent modality of ventilation. One may argue that more significant differences could have been seen if the intervention continued longer, particularly in the lower birth weight stratum. The study was designed to examine the role of PSV as one of the lung protective ventilatory strategies during the early course of mechanical ventilation, however, and this study did show that ELBW preterm infants at risk for ventilator-induced lung injury and BPD benefit most from faster weaning of the ventilatory support if PSV is added to SIMV.

Pressure support ventilation as an adjunct to volume-targeted synchronized intermittent mandatory ventilation

PSV seems to be an attractive adjunct to volume-controlled ventilation in infants who have reliable spontaneous respiratory drive. One such refinement is volume-assured pressure support, or VAPS, which incorporates inspiratory pressure support with conventional volume-assisted cycles. In this modality, the physician determines the pressure support level, peak flow, and a guaranteed tidal volume. If the patient demand is high relative to the peak flow and tidal volume settings, pressure augmentation functions similarly to PSV but guarantees the delivery of a minimal tidal volume by transitioning to a square wave flow pattern, increasing the inspiratory time, and ramping the pressure.

Several studies in newborn infants have shown that addition of volume guarantee (VG) to various neonatal patient-triggered ventilatory modes results in significant reduction in PIP and hence in $\overline{Paw}$ [26–28]. Abubakar and colleagues [26], in a short-term crossover study of 23 infants of gestational aged 31 ± 6 weeks who were in the recovery phase of RDS, reported that this reduction in PIP and $\overline{Paw}$ was maximum and less variable when VG was combined with PSV, because every breath was supported in PSV plus VG. PSV alone can lead to shorter Ti (inspiratory time) and thus provides better synchrony and smoother ventilation, which may further reduce $\overline{Paw}$ during PSV plus VG [19,26]. Similar observations were made by El-Moneim and colleagues [29] in a crossover trial comparing PSV plus VG with SIMV in 25 ventilated preterm infants in their weaning phase. Although the absolute decrease in pressure when switching between SIMV and PSV plus VG to provide constant V_T was small (probably because of mild lung disease in the study infants), the Ti, PIP, and $\overline{Paw}$ were always lower during PSV plus VG compared with SIMV. Hypocapnia can occur with PSV, however, because the ventilator is triggered with every spontaneous breath. Adding VG to PSV may fail to correct this problem, especially in infants who have strong respiratory drive who are approaching extubation. In the study by El-Moneim and colleagues [29], the hypocapnia seen soon after switching from SIMV to PSV plus VG resolved spontaneously toward the end of a 30-minute PSV plus VG ventilation period.

PSV in conjunction with synchronized volume-targeted ventilation has the potential to reduce ventilator-inflicted lung injury by allowing the infants to control the inspiration and limiting the pressure required to achieve the desired tidal volume, particularly during the acute phase of RDS following surfactant administration. This phase is characterized by dynamically changing functional residual capacity, compliance, resistance, and spontaneous respiratory effort.

In a small RCT [30], initial 24-hour ventilatory parameters were compared in two groups of 34 preterm very low birth weight infants managed by PSV with volume guarantee (PSV-VG) or SIMV after surfactant treatment of RDS. The use of PSV-VG as an initial ventilatory mode achieved accelerated weaning of peak inspiratory pressure and mean airway pressure compared with SIMV. After 24 hours, ventilation management was at the discretion of the attending neonatologists, and because of the subjectivity in how ventilators were set up and managed the benefit of faster weaning could not be adequately evaluated with respect to time to extubation and the incidence of chronic lung disease. By contrast, in another small but similar randomized crossover trial that enrolled 14 preterm infants (gestational age 34 ± 2, age at enrollment 49 ± 6 hours) who had uncomplicated RDS, minute ventilation was greater, and mean airway pressure was higher during 4 hours of PSV plus VG compared with SIMV [31]. This study is fraught with several problems regarding the design, data acquisition, and data interpretation [32].

All these short-term studies demonstrate that combining PSV with a volume-targeted mode of ventilation is feasible, safe, and well tolerated in premature infants, but evidence for benefits from well-controlled and adequately powered randomized studies focusing on longer-term outcomes is lacking.

Summary

PSV, one of the newest ventilatory modes, provides an inspiratory pressure boost during spontaneous breathing to overcome the imposed work of breathing. Currently, RCTs comparing PSV with the newer synchronized ventilatory modes remain limited, but all available data indicate that PSV is safe and well tolerated even when used in premature extremely low birth weight newborn infants. Preliminary application of PSV to the neonatal population shows great promise. Applications include weaning during volume-controlled ventilation and in conjunction with SIMV, ventilatory management of infants who have BPD who are unresponsive to conventional ventilatory strategies, and as a primary management strategy for RDS.

Clinical trials performed to date have demonstrated short-term safety and a physiologic proof of concept. Until further RCTs examine long-term outcomes, the decision to use PSV in neonates will continue to be based on the understanding of the concept and design characteristics of an inspiratory assist, a desire to achieve patient–ventilator synchrony and comfort, one's own experience with PSV, and the results of the short-term observational studies that show positive physiologic effects and improved short-term clinical outcomes.

References

[1] Kacmarek RM. Inspiratory pressure support: does it make a clinical difference? Intensive Care Med 1989;15(6):337–9.
[2] MacIntyre NR. Respiratory function during pressure support ventilation. Chest 1986;89(5): 677–83.
[3] Banner MJ, Kirby RR, MacIntyre NR. Patient and ventilator work of breathing and ventilatory muscle loads at different levels of pressure support ventilation. Chest 1991;100(2): 531–3.
[4] Tokioka H, Saito S, Kosaka F. Comparison of pressure support ventilation and assist control ventilation in patients with acute respiratory failure. Intensive Care Med 1989;15(6): 364–7.
[5] Stewart KG. Clinical evaluation of pressure support ventilation. Br J Anaesth 1989;63(3): 362–4.
[6] Valentine DD, Hammond MD, Downs JB, et al. Distribution of ventilation and perfusion with different modes of mechanical ventilation. Am Rev Respir Dis 1991;143(6):1262–6.
[7] Tokioka H, Saito S, Takahashi T, et al. Effectiveness of pressure support ventilation for mechanical ventilatory support in patients with status asthmaticus. Acta Anaesthesiol Scand 1992;36(1):5–9.
[8] Dries DJ, Kumar P, Mathru M, et al. Hemodynamic effects of pressure support ventilation in cardiac surgery patients. Am Surg 1991;57(2):122–5.
[9] Brochard L, Rauss A, Benito S, et al. Comparison of three methods of gradual withdrawal from ventilatory support during weaning from mechanical ventilation. Am J Respir Crit Care Med 1994;150(4):896–903.
[10] Esteban A, Frutos F, Tobin MJ, et al. A comparison of four methods of weaning patients from mechanical ventilation. Spanish Lung Failure Collaborative Group. N Engl J Med 1995;332(6):345–50.
[11] Butler R, Keenan SP, Inman KJ, et al. Is there a preferred technique for weaning the difficult-to-wean patient? A systematic review of the literature. Crit Care Med 1999;27(11):2331–6.
[12] Randolph AG, Wypij D, Venkataraman ST, et al. Pediatric Acute Lung Injury and Sepsis Investigators (PALISI) Network. Effect of mechanical ventilator weaning protocols on respiratory outcomes in infants and children: a randomized controlled trial. JAMA 2002; 288(20):2561–8.
[13] Quinn MW, de Boer RC, Ansari N, et al. Stress response and mode of ventilation in preterm infants. Arch Dis Child Fetal Neonatal Ed 1998;78(3):F195–8.
[14] Ramanathan R. Synchronized intermittent mandatory ventilation and pressure support: to sync or not to sync? Pressure support or no pressure support? J Perinatol 2005;25(Suppl 2): S23–5.

[15] Nicks JJ, Becker MA, Donn SM. Ventilatory management casebook. Bronchopulmonary dysplasias. Response to pressure support ventilation. J Perinatol 1994;14(6):495–7.

[16] Tokioka H, Nagano O, Ohta Y, et al. Pressure support ventilation augments spontaneous breathing with improved thoracoabdominal synchrony in neonates with congenital heart disease. Anesth Analg 1997;85(4):789–93.

[17] Heldt GP, McIlroy MB. Distortion of chest wall and work of diaphragm in preterm infants. J Appl Physiol 1987;62(1):164–9.

[18] Jubran A, Van de Graff WB, Tobin MJ. Variability of patient-ventilator interaction with pressure support ventilation in patients with chronic obstructive pulmonary disease. Am J Respir Crit Care Med 1995;152:129–36.

[19] Kapasi M, Fujino Y, Kirmse M, et al. Effort and work of breathing in neonates during assisted patient-triggered ventilation. Pediatr Crit Care Med 2001;2(1):9–16.

[20] Black JW, Grover BS. A hazard of pressure support ventilation. Chest 1988;93(2):333–5.

[21] Osorio W, Claure N, D'Ugard C, et al. Effects of pressure support during an acute reduction of synchronized intermittent mandatory ventilation in preterm infants. J Perinatol 2005; 25(6):412–6.

[22] Sinha SK, Donn SM, Gavey J, et al. Randomised trial of volume controlled versus time cycled, pressure limited ventilation in preterm infants with respiratory distress syndrome. Arch Dis Child Fetal Neonatal Ed 1997;77(3):F202–5.

[23] Keszler M. Pressure support ventilation and other approaches to overcome imposed work of breathing. Neoreviews 2006;7:e226–33.

[24] Sinha S, Donn SM. Feasibility of pressure support ventilation in low birth weight infants [abstract]. Joint meeting of the Irish Perinatal Society and the British Association of Perinatal Medicine. Dublin, Ireland, October 1, 1994.

[25] Reyes ZC, Claure N, Tauscher MK, et al. Randomized, controlled trial comparing synchronized intermittent mandatory ventilation and synchronized intermittent mandatory ventilation plus pressure support in preterm infants. Pediatrics 2006;118(4):1409–17.

[26] Abubakar KM, Keszler M. Patient-ventilator interactions in new modes of patient-triggered ventilation. Pediatr Pulmonol 2001;32:71–5.

[27] Cheema IU, Ahluwalia JS. Feasibility of tidal volume-guided ventilation in newborn infants: a randomized, crossover trial using the volume guarantee modality. Pediatrics 2001;107: 1323–8.

[28] Herrera CM, Gerhardt T, Everett R, et al. Randomized, crossover study of volume guarantee (VG) versus synchronized intermittent mandatory ventilation (SIMV) in very low birth weight (VLBW) infants recovering from respiratory failure. Pediatr Res 1999;45:304A.

[29] Abd El-Moneim ES, Fuerste HO, Krueger M, et al. Pressure support ventilation combined with volume guarantee versus synchronized intermittent mandatory ventilation: a pilot crossover trial in premature infants in their weaning phase. Pediatr Crit Care Med 2005; 6(3):286–92.

[30] Nafday Suhas M, Green Robert S, Lin Jing, et al. Is there an advantage of using pressure support ventilation with volume guarantee in the initial management of premature infants with respiratory distress syndrome? A pilot study. J Perinatol 2005;25:193–7.

[31] Olsen SL, Thibeault DW, Truog WE. Crossover trial comparing pressure support with synchronized intermittent mandatory ventilation. J Perinatol 2002;22:461–6.

[32] Keszler M, Abubakar KM, Mammel MC. Response to Olsen, et al. study comparing SIMV & PSV. J Perinatol 2003;23:434–5.

ELSEVIER
SAUNDERS

CLINICS IN
PERINATOLOGY

Clin Perinatol 34 (2007) 129–144

The Role of High-Frequency Ventilation in Neonates: Evidence-Based Recommendations

Andrea L. Lampland, MD[a],*,
Mark C. Mammel, MD[a,b]

[a]Division of Neonatology, Department of Pediatrics, University of Minnesota,
420 Delaware St. SE, Minneapolis, MN 55455, USA
[b]Infant Diagnostic & Research Center, Children's Hospital of Minnesota–St. Paul,
347 N. Smith Avenue, Rm. 505, St. Paul, MN 55102, USA

Respiratory failure in neonates, commonly defined as retention of carbon dioxide with a resultant decrease in the arterial blood pH and accompanied by hypoxemia, has multiple etiologies. It remains the most common complication of premature birth and the number one reason that neonates require assisted mechanical ventilation. Respiratory failure is a result of impaired pulmonary gas exchange mechanisms, such as can be seen with surfactant deficiency, atelectasis, or obstructive airway disease. Less common causes of respiratory failure may be a result of airway, musculature, or central nervous system abnormalities. The specific etiology of neonatal respiratory failure can, at times, be unclear and potentially multifactorial. Nonetheless, insights into the potential etiologies and pathophysiology of respiratory failure weigh heavily in the clinician's decisions regarding initiation of assisted mechanical ventilation.

Much progress has been made in the treatment of neonatal respiratory failure over the past few decades. In particular, antenatal steroids and exogenous surfactant replacement have decreased neonatal mortality and morbidity in premature infants [1–3]. However, lung injury and pulmonary morbidities secondary to mechanical ventilation remain an ongoing problem in the care of premature infants. Of most concern, chronic lung disease (CLD) develops in up to one third of preterm infants who have respiratory

* Corresponding author. Division of Neonatology, Department of Pediatrics, University of Minnesota, 420 Delaware St. SE, Minneapolis, MN 55455.
E-mail address: lampl002@umn.edu (A.L. Lampland).

0095-5108/07/$ - see front matter © 2007 Elsevier Inc. All rights reserved.
doi:10.1016/j.clp.2006.12.004
perinatology.theclinics.com

distress syndrome (RDS) who receive positive pressure mechanical ventilation [4]. Dilemmas still remain regarding optimization of both timing and mode of mechanical ventilation to decrease neonatal pulmonary morbidities.

High-frequency ventilation (HFV) is a form of mechanical ventilation that uses small tidal volumes and extremely rapid ventilator rates. It first came to the attention of the medical community during the 1970s, when a number of scattered reports appeared. Lunkenheimer and colleagues [5] reported the use of high-frequency oscillatory ventilation (HFOV) in apneic dogs, Sjöstrand [6] used high-frequency positive pressure ventilation in adults who have respiratory failure, and Carlon and colleagues [7] used a type of jet ventilation in adults who have bronchopleural fistula. Early reports of neonatal use came from Frantz and colleagues [8] in Boston, Massachussetts, and Pokora and colleagues [9] in St. Paul, Minnesota. In an attempt to clarify how it is possible to maintain pulmonary gas exchange when the tidal volumes used are often smaller than the anatomic dead space, Chang [10] described the multiple modes of gas transport that occur during HFV, including bulk convection, high-frequency "pendulluft," convective dispersion, Taylor-type dispersion, and molecular diffusion. There are various high-frequency ventilator designs, including HFOV, high-frequency jet ventilation (HFJV), as well as "mixed" forms of HFV (eg, flow interrupters, high-frequency positive pressure ventilation). In the United States, the most commonly used high-frequency ventilators include the SensorMedics 3100A (SensorMedics Inc., Yorba Linda, California), which provides HFOV; the LifePulse high-frequency jet ventilator (Bunnell Inc., Salt Lake City, Utah), which provides HFJV; and the Infant Star ventilator (InfraSonics Inc., San Diego, California), which is a high-frequency flow interrupter (HFFI).

Potential advantages of HFV over conventional mechanical ventilation (CMV) include the use of small tidal volumes, the ability to independently manage ventilation and oxygenation, and the safer use of mean airway pressure that is higher than that generally used during CMV [11]. Animal studies suggest that HFV works at lower proximal airway pressures than CMV, reduces ventilator-related lung injury, improves gas exchange in the face of air leaks, and decreases oxygen requirements [12–17]. Most causes of neonatal respiratory insufficiency requiring mechanical ventilation are amenable to treatment with HFV or CMV. For either technique to be successful, lung volumes need to be optimized for the underlying condition, and pressure exposures must likewise be similarly regulated. Only by the careful application of the chosen technique can ventilator-induced lung injury be avoided. The question remains, however: is one form of ventilation better than the other?

Despite the wealth of laboratory and clinical research on HFV, there are no established guidelines for prioritizing the use of HFV versus CMV in neonatal respiratory failure. Since 1997, approximately 25% of infants born at 1500 g or less reported to the Vermont–Oxford Network have been treated at some time with HFV [18]. Some clinicians choose to use HFV as the primary mode of mechanical ventilation for small infants. Others elect to only use HFV as a "rescue" method when CMV is failing. Most clinicians stand somewhere in the middle of this spectrum. This article is not a "how to" guide for the use of HFV. Rather, it reviews and evaluates the available literature to determine the evidence base for the use of HFV in neonatal respiratory failure.

Evidence review

An evidence review was performed to answer the following questions:

1. In the presence of acute neonatal respiratory failure or respiratory distress syndrome, does elective use of HFV provide benefit over the use of CMV?
2. In the presence of ongoing, severe neonatal respiratory failure, does the use of HFV as a rescue mode of ventilation provide benefit over the continued use of CMV?
3. Are there specific etiologies to neonatal respiratory failure in which HFV has been superior to CMV?

An electronic search of Medline and the Cochrane Database of Systematic Reviews was performed to identify relevant studies to these questions. The key words used for the search regarding the first two questions were high frequency ventilation (including high frequency oscillatory ventilation and high frequency jet ventilation) and respiratory insufficiency. The time frame searched was from 1985 to 2006, with limitation of studies related to the age range "birth to 23 months." The search produced the following number of citations: high frequency ventilation 657 articles, respiratory insufficiency 4090 articles, HFV and respiratory insufficiency 118 articles. Selected articles, in particular controlled clinical trials and meta-analyses, were reviewed and presented in this article regarding the current role of HFV in neonates.

Elective high-frequency ventilation

Literature review

To date, there have been 15 randomized controlled clinical trials of elective use of HFV versus CMV for the treatment of premature neonates who have respiratory insufficiency or RDS. One additional study compares the use of HFV versus CMV in term and near-term infants. These trials and their pulmonary outcomes are summarized in Table 1 [19–34]. The data from these 16 randomized controlled trials of HFV have yielded conflicting results. Five of the 16 trials demonstrated that early elective use of HFV improved pulmonary outcomes, in particular, decreased the incidence of

Table 1
Summary of randomized controlled trials of elective use of high-frequency ventilation versus conventional mechanical ventilation

References	Infants in trial	Eligibility criteria	Type of HFV	Pulmonary-related results
HiFi [19]	673	Respiratory failure, 750–2000 g	HFOV (Hummingbird, Senko Medical)	No difference in CLD or death. Increased air leaks in HFOV-treated group.
Carlo et al [20]	42	RDS, 1000–2000 g	HFJV (not stated)	No difference in death, air leaks, or CLD.
Clark et al [21]	83	RDS, <35 wk, ≤1750 g	HFOV (SensorMedics 3100A)	HFOV-only decreased CLD compared with CMV only. HFOV x 72 h followed by CMV did not decrease CLD.
Ogawa et al [22]	92	RDS, 750–2000 g	HFOV (Hummingbird, Senko Medical)	No difference in death, duration of mechanical ventilation, CLD, or air leaks.
Wiswell et al [23]	73	RDS, <33 wk, >500 g	HFJV (Bunnell Life Pulse)	No difference in air leaks, duration of mechanical ventilation, or CLD. Increased poor outcomes (grade 4 ICH, cystic PVL, or death) in HFJV group.
Gerstmann et al [24]	125	RDS, <35 wk	HFOV (SensorMedics 3100A)	HFOV decreased oxygen use, days on mechanical ventilation, and CLD. No difference in air leaks.
Keszler et al [25]	130	RDS, <36 wk, 700–1500 g	HFJV (Bunnell Life Pulse)	HFJV decreased oxygen use and CLD. No difference in air leaks.
Rettwitz-Volk et al [26]	96	RDS, <32 wk	HFOV (Stephan SHF 3000)	No difference in duration of mechanical ventilation, air leaks, CLD or death.
Plavka et al [27]	43	RDS, 500–1500 g	HFOV (SensorMedics 3100A)	HFOV reduced CLD. No difference in air leaks or duration of mechanical ventilation.

	N	Population	Device	Results
Thome et al [28]	284	RDS, ≥24–<30 wk	HFFI (Infant Star HFV)	HFFI was associated with more air leaks. No difference in duration of mechanical ventilation, death, or CLD.
Moriette et al [29]	273	RDS, 24–29 wk	HFOV (OHF1)	HFOV decreased need for surfactant. No difference in air leaks or CLD.
Courtney et al [30]	500	RDS, 601–1200 g, one dose of surfactant	HFOV (SensorMedics 3100A)	HFOV decreased age to extubation and CLD. No difference in death.
Johnson et al [31]	797	RDS, 23–28 wk	HFOV (Dräger Babylog 8000, SensorMedics 3100A, SLE 2000HFO)	No difference in CLD, air leaks, or death.
Van Reempts et al [32]	300	RDS, <32 wk	HFOV (SensorMedics 3100A) or HFFI (Infant Star HFV)	No difference in CLD, air leaks, duration of mechanical ventilation, or death.
Craft et al [33]	46	Respiratory insufficiency, 23–34 wk, <1000 g	HFFI (Infant Star HFV)	No difference in CLD, air leaks, duration of mechanical ventilation, or death.
Rojas et al [34]	119	Respiratory failure, >35 wk CGA, ≥1750 g	HFOV (SensorMedics 3100A)	No difference in CLD, air leaks, duration of mechanical ventilation, or death.

Abbreviations: CGA, corrected gestational age; ICH, intracranial hemorrhage; PVL, periventricular leukomalacia.

chronic lung disease, as compared with CMV [21,24,25,27,30]. The 11 remaining trials showed no difference in pulmonary outcomes when using HFV versus CMV [19,20,22,23,26,28,29,31–34]. Differences in high-frequency ventilators, ventilation strategies, definitions of chronic lung disease, study populations, and study center experiences over time, as well as the inability to blind the treatment intervention, may be the derivation of such incongruent results regarding early use of HFV versus CMV. Likewise, some of the studies were conducted before routine use of exogenous surfactant. Nonetheless, HFV is routinely used in many neonatal ICUs, and we need to glean as much knowledge as possible from the current body of evidence in the literature.

The HiFi trial [19], published in 1989, was the first controlled trial of HFV versus CMV in neonates and the second largest study of its kind to date. In the HFV group, the Hummingbird HFOV (Metran Co. Ltd., Saitama, Japan) was used at mean airway pressures comparable to those delivered by CMV. The study demonstrated no significant differences in the incidence of death (HFV, 18%; CMV, 17%) or chronic lung disease (HFV, 40%; CMV, 41%), defined as oxygen requirement and abnormal chest radiographic findings at 28 days between the two groups. Of concern, the study found significantly increased air leaks and severe intracranial pathology, including grade 3 and 4 intracranial hemorrhage and periventricular leukomalacia (PVL), in the HFV group. In a smaller study using the same Hummingbird HFOV and the same criteria for defining chronic lung disease but implementing a lung volume recruitment strategy, Ogawa and colleagues [22] demonstrated no significant differences in death or chronic lung disease in HFV- versus CMV-treated groups. In contrast to the HiFi study, however, this study did not show any significant difference is air leaks or severe intracranial pathology between the groups.

Although small in size, two studies by Carlo and colleagues [20] and Wiswell and colleagues [23] comparing HFV delivered by a HFJV versus CMV did not demonstrate any significant differences in pulmonary outcomes or mortality between each group. The studies did have conflicting results regarding intracranial pathology. Carlo and colleagues demonstrated no significant difference in the incidence of grade 2 through 4 intraventricular hemorrhage (IVH) between the two groups, whereas Wiswell and colleagues showed significantly more severe intracranial pathology (grade 3–4 IVH and PVL) in those treated with HFJV.

Ventilation with high-frequency flow interrupters versus CMV has been looked at in a large trial of 284 patients by Thome and colleagues [28] in 1999, and in a smaller, more recent study, the Sy-Fi study, by Craft and colleagues [33]. Thome's study included babies 24 to 30 weeks, whereas the Sy-Fi study included similarly aged babies but added a weight criterion of less than 1000 g. Both studies demonstrated no difference in chronic lung disease, mortality, or severe IVH. Both demonstrated increased air leaks in the HFFI-treated groups. In the Sy-Fi study, however, it was a select group of infants, those treated with HFFI and weighing more (751–1000 g), that had a higher incidence of air leaks.

The vast majority of controlled trials of HFV versus CMV have employed HFOVs. However, the types of oscillator, some of which are not commercially available in the United States, varied from study to study, and one must be cognizant of this variable when comparing studies. In the largest trial of HFV versus CMV to date, Johnson and colleagues [31] included 797 preterm infants and used multiple different types of HFOV in the HFV arm. This trial demonstrated no difference in air leaks, CLD, or death in the HFV-treated group compared with the CMV-treated group. Unlike the concerning findings of the initial large HiFi study, Johnson and colleagues did not demonstrate any differences in severe IVH or PVL between the two treatment groups. Similarly, trials conducted by Rettwitz-Volk and colleagues [26] and Moriette and colleagues [29], using oscillators that are not commercially available in the United States, did not document an advantage of HFOV over CMV, with the exception of decreased exogenous surfactant requirements in the HFOV arm of the Moriette trial. Lastly, a recent prospective controlled trial of HFV versus CMV by Van Reempts and colleagues [32] revealed information on short-term endpoints as well as long-term follow-up results. They employed either HFOV or HFFI to provide HFV. The trial demonstrated no difference in duration of ventilation, air leaks, CLD, or mortality between the HFV and CMV groups. Looking at short- and long-term neurologic findings, they found no differences in the incidence of severe intracranial hemorrhage, PVL, or in the scores of more long-term assessment of motor and cognitive function at approximately 1 year of age.

To date, five controlled trials of HFV versus CMV have shown a benefit in pulmonary outcomes in the HFV groups. Favorable pulmonary results in the HFV-treated groups have occurred in less than one third of the total number of controlled trials of HFV versus CMV, and it is worth noting that most of these "positive" trials used HFOV (SensorMedics 3100A) as the means to provide HFV. Clark and colleagues [21] published the first positive trial in 1992. This single center study had three arms: HFOV only, HFOV for 72 hours followed by CMV, and CMV only. Babies in the HFOV-only arm had a decreased incidence of CLD. None of the three groups differed significantly in the incidence of air leaks, IVH, or death. Subsequently, Gerstmann and colleagues [24], in a multicenter controlled trial, demonstrated similar results of beneficial pulmonary outcomes with HFV, including a decreased need for multiple doses of surfactant and decreased incidence of CLD. Plavka and colleagues [27], in a smaller, single-center study, concluded similar results of decreased need for exogenous surfactant and decreased CLD in HFOV-treated babies. By far the most notable of the positive trials comes from Courtney and colleagues [30] and the Neonatal Ventilation Study Group. They published the largest controlled trial to date that demonstrates a benefit of HFV in pulmonary outcomes. This study included 500 preterm neonates who received at least one dose of surfactant. The neonates randomized to the HFOV arm had significantly fewer days of mechanical ventilation as well as a decreased incidence of CLD compared with those treated with CMV. There was no difference in mortality, IVH, or PVL between the groups.

There is only one controlled trial of HFJV versus CMV that has ever demonstrated a beneficial pulmonary effect from using early, elective HFJV. Keszler and colleagues [25], in a multicenter controlled trial of 130 babies who had RDS, demonstrated a decreased incidence of CLD at 36 weeks corrected gestational age, as well as a decreased need for home oxygen therapy in the HFJV-treated group. Furthermore, there were no differences in air leaks, IVH, or death between the two groups.

Evidence-based recommendations

There is no evidence from the authors' current review of the literature or other meta-analyses that elective use of HFV, in the form of HFOV or HFFI, provides any greater benefit to premature infants who have RDS than CMV [35]. The data are limited and the results are mixed as to whether HFJV may reduce the incidence of CLD [36]. At this time, preferential use of HFV as the initial mode of ventilation to treat premature infants who have RDS is not supported.

Gaps in knowledge

Ventilation strategies play a potentially significant role in pulmonary outcomes. There are no standardized criteria for the optimal use of HFV, nor are there sufficient data to determine the best techniques for lung recruitment. Similarly, though recruitment and maintenance of lung volume is an important component of treatment for many conditions, there are no easy-to-use techniques for accurate clinical measurement of lung volumes at the bedside. Finally, the use of so-called "high-volume ventilation strategies" versus "low-volume ventilation strategies" is incompletely defined, and the issue of which ventilator to use to provide HFV is unknown. In the same light, standardized strategies have not been defined for the optimal use of CMV, which today has many different ventilation modes and modalities available for clinical use. Lastly, and perhaps most important, long-term neurodevelopmental outcomes are of particular interest to physicians treating premature infants; these are lacking in most published studies.

Rescue high-frequency ventilation

Literature review

The body of literature regarding the use of HFV as a rescue technique is small and incomplete. In particular, there are only two controlled trials to date that explore this issue in premature infants who have severe respiratory distress. If controlled trials comparing rescue HFV versus CMV in term and near-term infants are included, the total number of studies only increases to four. These trials and their pulmonary outcomes are summarized in Table 2 [37–40].

The HIFO trial investigated whether the use of rescue HFOV provides any benefit over continued CMV in preterm infants who have severe respiratory insufficiency, in particular with regard to pulmonary air leaks [38]. The HIFO trial randomized 176 preterm infants (<35 weeks, >500 g) who had severe respiratory distress, and had or were at increased risk of developing pulmonary air leak to HFOV versus continued CMV. This trial demonstrated a reduction in new pulmonary air leaks in the HFOV arm; however, there was no significant difference in the incidence of ongoing pulmonary interstitial emphysema, pneumomediastinum, or pneumothorax overall. There was also no difference in duration of mechanical ventilation or death between the two groups. IVH rates were increased in the HFOV-treated group compared with the CMV-treated group. This is a potentially worrisome finding, and unfortunately, there is no long-term neurologic or developmental follow-up described in this study.

In a more select population, Keszler and colleagues [37] randomized 144 preterm infants (<35 weeks, ≥750 g and <2000 g) who had severe respiratory failure and pulmonary interstitial emphysema to ventilation with the Bunnell HFJV device versus continued CMV at high rates. The study did allow for crossover if an infant met criteria for failure of the initially allocated ventilation mode. A significant number of patients in both groups met failure criteria (39% HFJV, 63% CMV) and crossed over to the alternate ventilation strategy. This being said, the patients treated with HFJV had more rapid improvement of their pulmonary interstitial emphysema. However, there were no differences in chronic lung disease, new air leaks, severe IVH, or mortality between the two groups. When the crossover population was excluded, the study demonstrated a lower mortality rate in the HFJV-treated group compared with the CMV-treated group.

The two aforementioned controlled studies of rescue HFV versus CMV in preterm infants were completed at a time when exogenous surfactant and antenatal steroids were not necessarily administered on a routine basis. Therefore, the generalization of specific results to today's neonatal ICU population can potentially be called into question. The controlled studies of rescue HFV versus CMV in term or near-term infants by Clark and colleagues [39] and Engle and colleagues [40] are somewhat more applicable because they were performed more recently, and the infants studied are of a gestational age that antenatal steroids and exogenous surfactant are not obligatory. Nonetheless, since the time of their publication, exogenous surfactant and other interventions, such as inhaled nitric oxide (iNO), are used with increasing frequency and are not accounted for in these studies.

Clark and colleagues [39] randomized 79 term or near-term infants (>34 weeks, ≥2000 g) who had severe respiratory failure from various etiologies (meconium aspiration, RDS, pneumonia, congenital diaphragmatic hernia,

Table 2
Summary of randomized controlled trials of rescue use of high-frequency ventilation versus conventional mechanical ventilation

References	Infants in trial	Eligibility criteria	Type of HFV	Pulmonary-related results
Keszler et al [37]	144	Pulmonary interstitial emphysema on CMV, ≥750 g	HFJV (Bunnell Life Pulse)	Increased treatment success in HFJV group. Decreased mortality in HFJV group is crossover excluded. No difference in CLD, new air leaks, airway obstruction, or necrotizing tracheobronchitis.
HIFO Study Group [38]	176	Severe RDS, ≥500 g, <48 h old	HFOV (SensorMedics 3100A)	Decreased new air leaks in HFOV group. No difference in ongoing air leak syndrome, duration of mechanical ventilation, or death.
Clark et al [39]	79	Severe respiratory failure, >34 wk, ≥2000 g, <14 d old	HFOV (SensorMedics 3100A)	Improved gas exchange and increased treatment success in HFOV group. No difference in CLD, air leaks, duration of mechanical ventilation, need for ECMO, or death.
Engle et al [40]	24	Severe respiratory failure and pulmonary hypertension, ≥35 wk, >2000 g	HFJV (Bunnell Life Pulse)	Improved gas exchange in HFJV group. No difference in CLD, air leaks, duration of mechanical ventilation, need for ECMO, or death.

Abbreviation: ECMO, extracorporeal membrane oxygenation.

other) to HFOV versus continued CMV. The average age at randomization was 37 to 40 hours, and crossover to the alternate form of ventilation was allowed if preset criteria for treatment failure were achieved. The study demonstrated improved gas exchange and less treatment failure with HFOV, both in the patients initially allocated to rescue HFOV as well as in those that failed continued CMV and crossed over to HFOV. There was no difference in the incidence of chronic lung disease, IVH, or death between the two groups.

Engle and colleagues [40] randomized a more specific population of term and near-term infants (≥ 35 weeks, >2000 g) who had severe persistent pulmonary hypertension to HFJV versus CMV. The average age at randomization was 22 to 25 hours and crossover for treatment failure was not allowed in this study, because those who failed their allocated form of ventilation were referred for extracorporeal membrane oxygenation (ECMO). In this study, the HFJV-treated patients had improved oxygenation and ventilation versus the CMV-treated group; however, there were no long-term differences in the duration of mechanical ventilation or the incidence of chronic lung disease, air leaks, IVH, patients requiring ECMO, or death.

Evidence-based recommendations

Although limited in nature, there is no evidence from the authors' current review of the randomized controlled trials or other meta-analyses that use of rescue HFV provides any long-term benefit over continued CMV in the preterm, near-term, or term patient who has respiratory failure [41–43].

Gaps in knowledge

Although there is a significant amount of data from nonrandomized uncontrolled trials regarding the use of rescue HFV in babies who have an inadequate response to CMV, such as that by Davis and colleagues [44], few randomized controlled trials of HFV versus CMV in conditions other than acute RDS in the preterm infant exist. Similarly, the few randomized trials that have been published regarding rescue HFV were performed when the administration of exogenous surfactant and antenatal steroids were not the norm. Current randomized clinical trials of rescue HFV are necessary.

High-frequency ventilation for conditions other than respiratory distress syndrome—management of bronchopleural or tracheoesophageal fistula, and high-frequency ventilation plus inhaled nitric oxide

Literature review

Because of the low occurrence rates of bronchopleural and tracheo-esophageal fistulas in neonates, there are no randomized controlled trials evaluating their management with HFV versus CMV. However, a few studies have formally evaluated the amount of air leak through these types of fistulas using HFV versus CMV. In the management of infants who had bronchopleural fistula, Gonzales and colleagues [45] showed a decrease in chest tube air leak when using HFJV versus CMV. Goldberg and colleagues [46] and Donn and colleagues [47] reported similar experiences in managing infants who had tracheoesophageal fistulas with HFJV. Furthermore, case reports, such as that by Bloom and colleagues [48], and animal studies, such as that by Orlando and colleagues [49], relay findings of an observed benefit to the use of HFV in the ventilatory stabilization of patients who have tracheoesophageal or bronchopleural fistula.

Another common use for HFV in the neonatal population is in conjunction with iNO for severe hypoxemic respiratory failure, often as a result of persistent pulmonary hypertension. In a randomized controlled trial, Kinsella and colleagues [50] looked at the effects of combining HFOV with iNO compared with either therapy used alone in infants who have persistent pulmonary hypertension. This study enrolled 205 neonates who had pulmonary hypertension from various underlying etiologies and demonstrated maximal treatment success (better arterial oxygenation) with the simultaneous use of HFOV and iNO. When looking at the premature population, Schreiber and colleagues [51] did not find such a benefit from ventilation modality. They enrolled 207 infants born at less than 34 weeks gestation into a randomized, double-blind, controlled study of iNO and differing ventilation strategies with CMV versus HFOV. There was no difference in pulmonary outcomes or death directly related to ventilation mode. In a randomized study of pediatric patients who had hypoxemic respiratory failure, Dobyns and colleagues [52] found similar results to Kinsella's study with maximally improved oxygenation when using the combination of HFOV plus iNO as compared with HFOV alone, CMV plus iNO, or CMV alone. Although iNO is a new therapy and its potential synergy with HFV is similarly rather new, bench research further confirmed adequate and accurate delivery of iNO with both the HFOV and HFJV systems [53,54].

Evidence-based recommendations

Review of the literature supports the use of HFV with iNO to maximize oxygenation and treatment effects in hypoxemic respiratory failure, in particular in babies who have pulmonary hypertension. The current literature lacks any randomized trials to support the use of HFV over CMV in the treatment bronchopleural or tracheoesophageal fistula. That being said, the data do merit consideration, as the use of HFV in this population appears to diminish the amount of continuous air leak and improve patient stabilization.

Gaps in knowledge

Ideally, randomized trials are needed to elucidate the optimal ventilatory strategy in infants who have bronchopleural or tracheoesophageal fistula. However, because of the small number of patients who have these problems, it is unlikely that a randomized controlled trial will ever be feasible.

Summary

High-frequency ventilation is a form of mechanical ventilation that uses small tidal volumes and extremely rapid ventilator rates. It allows for pulmonary gas exchange at lower mean airway pressures than conventional mechanical ventilation. When HFV was first introduced on the menu of respiratory therapies for sick babies, hope abounded that HFV would be the universal remedy for most forms of neonatal respiratory insufficiency. In particular, clinicians were optimistic that HFV could be particularly useful in decreasing the incidence of chronic lung disease of prematurity. After almost 20 years of data gathering, this does not appear to be the case. When looked at as a whole, the currently available randomized controlled trials comparing HFV versus CMV have not demonstrated any clear benefit of HFV either as a primary mode or as a rescue mode of ventilation in neonates who have respiratory insufficiency. However, the current literature does support the preferential use of HFV over CMV in conjunction with iNO to maximize oxygenation in hypoxemic respiratory failure, in particular, as a result of persistent pulmonary hypertension.

Clearly, HFV has become a reliable and useful addition to the various modes of mechanical ventilation in neonates. Nonetheless, as most causes of neonatal respiratory insufficiency requiring mechanical ventilation are amenable to treatment with HFV or CMV, clinical judgment still dictates the choice of one form or the other, because the high-quality evidence currently available is still inconclusive. Ongoing studies will ideally elucidate the optimal lung volume and ventilatory strategy for specific disease states as well as provide clinicians with long-term follow-up data regarding neurologic and developmental outcomes of children treated with the various forms of ventilation.

References

[1] Liggins GC, Howie RN. A controlled trial of antepartum glucocorticoid treatment for prevention of the respiratory distress syndrome in premature infants. Pediatrics 1972;50:515–25.
[2] Crowley PA. Antenatal corticosteroid therapy: a meta-analysis of the randomized trials, 1972 to 1994. Am J Obstet Gynecol 1995;173:322–35.
[3] Soll RF. Prophylactic natural surfactant extract for preventing morbidity and mortality in preterm infants. Cochrane Database Syst Rev 2000;2:CD000511.
[4] Smith VC, Zupancic JA, McCormick MC, et al. Trends in severe bronchopulmonary dysplasia between 1994 and 2002. J Pediatr 2005;146:469–73.

[5] Lunkenheimer PP, Rafflenbeul W, Keller H. Application of transtracheal pressure oscillations as a modification of "diffusion respiration." Br J Anaesth 1972;44:627–8

[6] Sjostrand U. Summary of experimental and clinical features of high-frequency positive-pressure ventilation-HFPPV. Acta Anaesthesiol Scand Suppl 1977;64:55–68.

[7] Carlon GC, Ray C Jr, Klain M, et al. High-frequency positive-pressure ventilation in management of a patient with bronchopleural fistula. Anesthesiology 1980;52:160–2.

[8] Frantz ID 3rd, Werthammer J, Stark AR. High-frequency ventilation in premature infants with lung disease: adequate gas exchange at low tracheal pressure. Pediatrics 1983;14:483–8.

[9] Pokora T, Bing DR, Mammel MC, et al. Neonatal high-frequency jet ventilation. Pediatrics 1983;72:27–32.

[10] Chang HK. Mechanisms of gas transport during ventilation by high-frequency oscillation. J Appl Physiol 1984;56:553–63.

[11] Bunnell JB. High-frequency ventilation: general concepts. In: Donn SM, Sinha SK, editors. Neonatal respiratory care. 2nd edition. Philadelphia: Mosby, Inc.; 2006. p. 222–30.

[12] Boros SJ, Mammel MC, Coleman JM, et al. Comparison of high-frequency oscillatory ventilation and high-frequency jet ventilation in cats with normal lungs. Pediatr Pulmonol 1989;7:35–41.

[13] Thompson WK, Marchak BE, Froese AB, et al. High frequency oscillation compared with standard ventilation in pulmonary injury model. J Appl Physiol 1982;52:543–8.

[14] Bell RE, Kuehl TJ, Coalson JJ, et al. High-frequency ventilation compared to conventional positive-pressure ventilation in the treatment of hyaline membrane disease in primates. Crit Care Med 1984;12:764–8.

[15] Jackson JC, Truog WE, Standaert TA, et al. Effect of high-frequency ventilation on the development of alveolar edema in premature monkeys at risk for hyaline membrane disease. Am Rev Respir Dis 1991;143:865–71.

[16] Carlon GC, Ray C, Miodownik S, et al. Physiologic implications of high frequency jet ventilation techniques. Crit Care Med 1983;11:508–14.

[17] Lucking SE, Fields AI, Mahfood S, et al. High-frequency ventilation versus conventional ventilation in dogs with right ventricular dysfunction. Crit Care Med 1986;14:798–801.

[18] Horbar JD, Carpenter JH, Kenny M, editors. Vermont Oxford network annual database summaries 1997-2005. Burlington (VT): Vermont Oxford Network: 1998–2006.

[19] HiFi Study Group. High-frequency oscillatory ventilation compared with conventional mechanical ventilation in the treatment of respiratory failure in preterm infants. N Engl J Med 1989;320:88–93.

[20] Carlo WA, Siner B, Chatburn RL, et al. Early randomized intervention with high-frequency jet ventilation in respiratory distress syndrome. J Pediatr 1990;117:765–70.

[21] Clark RH, Gerstmann DR, Null DM, et al. Prospective randomized comparison of high-frequency oscillatory and conventional ventilation in respiratory distress syndrome. Pediatrics 1992;89:5–12.

[22] Ogawa Y, Miyasaka Y, Kawano T, et al. A multicenter randomized trial of high frequency oscillatory ventilation as compared with conventional mechanical ventilation in preterm infants with respiratory failure. Early Hum Dev 1993;32:1–10.

[23] Wiswell TE, Graziani LJ, Kornhauser MS, et al. High-frequency jet ventilation in the early management of respiratory distress syndrome is associated with a greater risk for adverse outcomes. Pediatrics 1996;98:1035–43.

[24] Gerstmann DR, Minton SD, Stoddard RA, et al. The provo multicenter early high-frequency oscillatory ventilation trial: improved pulmonary and clinical outcome in respiratory distress syndrome. Pediatrics 1996;98:1044–57.

[25] Keszler M, Modanlou HD, Brudno DS, et al. Multicenter controlled clinical trial of high-frequency jet ventilation in preterm infants with uncomplicated respiratory distress syndrome. Pediatrics 1997;100:593–9.

[26] Rettwitz-Volk W, Veldman A, Roth B, et al. A prospective, randomized, multicenter trial of high-frequency oscillatory ventilation compared with conventional ventilation in preterm infants with respiratory distress syndrome receiving surfactant. J Pediatr 1998; 132:249–54.

[27] Plavka R, Kopecky P, Sebron V, et al. A prospective randomized comparison of conventional mechanical ventilation and very early high frequency oscillatory ventilation in extremely premature newborns with respiratory distress syndrome. Intensive Care Med 1999;25:68–75.

[28] Thome U, Kossel H, Lipowsky G, et al. Randomized comparison of high-frequency ventilation with high-rate intermittent positive pressure ventilation in preterm infants with respiratory failure. J Pediatr 1999;135:39–46.

[29] Moriette G, Paris-Llado J, Walti H, et al. Prospective randomized multicenter comparison of high-frequency oscillatory ventilation and conventional ventilation in preterm infants of less than 30 weeks with respiratory distress syndrome. Pediatrics 2001;107:363–72.

[30] Courtney SE, Durand DJ, Asselin JM, et al. High-frequency oscillatory ventilation versus conventional mechanical ventilation for very-low-birth-weight infants. N Engl J Med 2002;347:643–52.

[31] Johnson AH, Peacock JL, Greenough A, et al. High-frequency oscillatory ventilation for the prevention of chronic lung disease of prematurity. N Engl J Med 2002;347:633–42.

[32] Van Reempts P, Borstlap C, Laroche S, et al. Early use of high frequency ventilation in the premature neonate. Eur J Pediatr 2003;162:219–26.

[33] Craft AP, Bhandari V, Finer NN. The Sy-Fi study: a randomized prospective trial of synchronized intermittent mandatory ventilation versus a high-frequency flow interrupter in infants less than 1000 g. J Perinatol 2003;23:14–9.

[34] Rojas MA, Lozano JM, Rojas MX, et al. Randomized, multicenter trial of conventional ventilation versus high-frequency oscillatory ventilation for the early management of respiratory failure in term or near-term infants in Colombia. J Perinatol 2005;25:720–4.

[35] Henderson-Smart DJ, Bhuta T, Cools F, et al. Elective high frequency oscillatory ventilation versus conventional ventilation for acute pulmonary dysfunction in preterm infants. Cochrane Database Syst Rev 2003;4:CD000104.

[36] Bhuta T, Henderson-Smart DJ. Elective high frequency jet ventilation versus conventional ventilation for respiratory distress syndrome in preterm infants. Cochrane Database Syst Rev 1998;2:CD000328.

[37] Keszler M, Donn SM, Bucciarelli RL, et al. Multicenter controlled trial comparing high-frequency jet ventilation and conventional mechanical ventilation in newborn infants with pulmonary interstitial emphysema. J Pediatr 1991;119:85–93.

[38] HIFO Study Group. Randomized study of high-frequency oscillatory ventilation in infants with severe respiratory distress syndrome. J Pediatr 1993;122:609–19.

[39] Clark RH, Yoder BA, Sell MS. Prospective, randomized comparison of high-frequency oscillation and conventional ventilation in candidates for extracorporeal membrane oxygenation. J Pediatr 1993;124:447–54.

[40] Engle WA, Yoder MC, Andreoli SP, et al. Controlled prospective randomized comparison of high-frequency jet ventilation and conventional ventilation in neonates with respiratory failure and persistent pulmonary hypertension. J Perinatol 1997;17:3–9.

[41] Bhuta T, Henderson-Smart DJ. Rescue high-frequency oscillatory ventilation versus conventional ventilation for pulmonary dysfunction in preterm infants. Cochrane Database Syst Rev 1998;2:CD000438.

[42] Joshi VH, Bhuta T. Rescue high frequency jet ventilation versus conventional ventilation for severe pulmonary dysfunction in preterm infants. Cochrane Database Syst Rev 2006;1: CD000437.

[43] Bhuta T, Clark RH, Henderson-Smart DJ. Rescue high frequency oscillatory ventilation vs. conventional ventilation for infants with severe pulmonary dysfunction born at or near term. Cochrane Database Syst Rev 2001;1:CD002974.

[44] Davis JM, Richter SE, Kendig JW, et al. High-frequency jet ventilation and surfactant treatment of newborns with severe respiratory failure. Pediatr Pulmonol 1992;13:108–12.

[45] Gonzalez F, Harris T, Black P, et al. Decreased gas flow through pneumothoraces in neonates receiving high-frequency jet versus conventional ventilation. J Pediatr 1987;110: 464–6.

[46] Goldberg L, Marmon L, Keszler M. High-frequency jet ventilation decreases flow through tracheo-esophageal fistula. Crit Care Med 1992;20:547–50.

[47] Donn SM, Zak LK, Bozynski ME, et al. Use of high-frequency jet ventilation in the management of congenital tracheoesophageal fistula associated with respiratory distress syndrome. J Pediatr Surg 1990;25:1219–21.

[48] Bloom BT, Delmore P, Park YI, et al. Respiratory distress syndrome and tracheoesophageal fistula: management with high-frequency ventilation. Crit Care Med 1990;18:447–8.

[49] Orlando R, Gluck EH, Cohen M, et al. Ultra-high-frequency jet ventilation in a broncho-pleural fistula model. Arch Surg 1988;123:591–3.

[50] Kinsella JP, Truog WE, Walsh WF, et al. Randomized, multicenter trial of inhaled nitric oxide and high-frequency oscillatory ventilation in severe, persistent pulmonary hypertension of the newborn. J Pediatr 1997;131:55–62.

[51] Schreiber MD, Gin-Mestan K, Marks JD, et al. Inhaled nitric oxide in premature infants with respiratory distress syndrome. N Engl J Med 2003;349:2099–107.

[52] Dobyns EL, Anas NG, Fortenberry JD, et al. Interactive effects of high-frequency oscillatory ventilation and inhaled nitric oxide in acute hypoxemic respiratory failure in pediatrics. Crit Care Med 2002;30:2425–9.

[53] Platt DR, Swanton D, Blackney D. Inhaled nitric oxide (iNO) delivery with high-frequency jet ventilation (HFJV). J Perinatol 2003;23:387–91.

[54] Fujino Y, Kacmarek RM, Hess DR. Nitric oxide delivery during high-frequency oscillatory ventilation. Respir Care 2000;45:1097–104.

CLINICS IN
PERINATOLOGY

ELSEVIER
SAUNDERS

Clin Perinatol 34 (2007) 145–177

Animal-Derived Surfactants Versus Past and Current Synthetic Surfactants: Current Status

Fernando Moya, MD[a,b,c,]*,
Andrés Maturana, MD, MSc[d,e]

[a]Department of Neonatology, New Hanover Regional Medical Center
and Coastal Area Health Education Center, 2131 South 17th Street,
Suite 405, Wilmington, NC 28402, USA
[b]University of North Carolina, Chapel Hill, NC 27599, USA
[c]Discovery Laboratories, Warrington, PA 18976, USA
[d]Servicio de Neonatologia, Clinica Alemana, Vitacura 5951, Santiago, Chile
[e]School of Medicine, Universidad del Desarrollo, Santiago, Chile

Administration of exogenous surfactant is one of the most well-studied therapies in neonatology. Furthermore, there is a good understanding of the mechanisms involved in the action of surfactant [1]. Multiple well-conducted clinical trials have demonstrated that its use in neonates at risk for respiratory distress syndrome (RDS), or who develop this form of lung disease, results in improvement in survival and a reduction in the occurrence of air leaks [2–4]. No decreases in complications of prematurity, such as bronchopulmonary dysplasia (BPD), intraventricular hemorrhage (IVH), retinopathy of prematurity (ROP), or necrotizing enterocolitis (NEC), have been consistently reported with this therapy, however. There are many surfactants currently available; no two are alike. The preparations most widely studied or used in neonates in the United States and Europe over the past decade are listed in Table 1. Based on their components, these can be grouped into the following families: synthetic surfactants that contain only phospholipids with no surfactant proteins (Exosurf [GlaxoSmithKline, Brentford, UK] and Pumactant [Britannia Pharmaceutical, Redhill, Surrey, UK]), animal-derived surfactants that contain phospholipids and variable amounts of surfactant proteins B (SP-B) and C (SP-C) (Survanta [Ross Products Division, Abbott Laboratories, Columbus, Ohio],

* Corresponding author. Department of Neonatology, New Hanover Regional Medical Center and Coastal Area Health Education Center, 2131 South 17th Street, Suite 405, Wilmington, NC 28402.
E-mail address: fernando.moya@coastalahec.org (F. Moya).

Table 1
Main characteristics of surfactants used in neonates

Surfactant	Family	Main phospholipids	Proteins	Phospholipid concentration	Suggested dose	Phospholipid per dose
Exosurf	Synthetic	DPPC	No	13.5 mg/mL	5 mL/kg	67.5 mg/kg
Pumactant	Synthetic	DPPC, PG	No	40 mg/mL	1.2 mL/kg	100 mg/kg
Survanta	Animal-derived (bovine)	DPPC, PG	Some SP-B and SP-C	25 mg/mL	4 mL/kg	100 mg/kg
Infasurf	Animal-derived (bovine)	DPPC, PG	SP-B and SP-C	35 mg/mL	3 mL/kg	105 mg/kg
Curosurf	Animal-derived (porcine)	DPPC, PG	SP-B and SP-C	80 mg/mL	2.5 mL/kg and 1.25 mL/kg	200 mg/kg or 100 mg/kg
Alveofact	Animal-derived (bovine)	DPPC, PG	SP-B and SP-C	40 mg/mL	1.2 mL/kg	50 mg/kg
Surfaxin	Peptide-containing synthetic	DPPC, POPG	KL_4 peptide as SP-B	30 mg/mL	5.8 mL/kg	175 mg/kg

Abbreviations: DPPC, dipalmitoylphosphatidylcholine; PG, phosphatidylglycerol; POPG, palmitoyloleylphosphatidylglycerol; SP-B, surfactant protein B; SP-C, surfactant protein C.

Infasurf [Forest Laboratories, Inc., St. Louis, Missouri], Curosurf [Chiesi Farmaceutici, Parma, Italy], and Alveofact [Boehringer Ingelheim, Ingelheim, Germany]), and a new generation of peptide-containing synthetic surfactants that have incorporated synthetic peptides modeled after SP-B or SP-C into mixtures of phospholipids (Surfaxin [Discovery Laboratories, Warrington, Pennsylvania] and Venticute [Nycomed, Roskilde, Denmark]). Only Surfaxin has been studied in neonates thus far. There are other less studied or used surfactants that are not addressed in this review [4].

Over the past 10 to 15 years, many trials comparing different surfactants have been reported [4–14]. A systematic review of 11 trials (9 published in full and 2 in abstract form) comparing synthetic and animal-derived surfactants reported that both types are beneficial for prevention and treatment of RDS. It also concluded that the use of animal-derived surfactants led to further reductions in mortality, a lower occurrence of pneumothorax, and faster weaning compared with synthetic surfactants [5]. All but one of the studies included in this review used surfactant for treatment of RDS. The synthetic surfactant group included primarily studies using Exosurf and only 1 trial of Pumactant, whereas the animal-derived group was represented by 7 trials of Survanta, two studies of Infasurf, and two studies that used Curosurf. A shortcoming of this review relates to the fact that all surfactants compared have different compositions, doses, and recommended frequencies of administration. Furthermore, there were important differences between trials in terms of study design, populations studied, and primary outcomes. There have been many other trials that have compared animal-derived surfactants and the newer generation of peptide-containing synthetic surfactants. To date, no detailed analysis of head-to-head comparisons of the various surfactant preparations has been conducted.

The goal of this review is to critically examine the evidence from comparison trials of various surfactant preparations, with special emphasis on comparisons of animal-derived surfactants versus previous synthetic surfactants and also versus the new generation of peptide-containing synthetic surfactants. Intentionally, this review only includes data from published clinical trials that have been subjected to the peer review process. Data available from abstracts or other non–peer-reviewed communications could not be reliably verified, even after an attempt was made to contact the authors. Furthermore, it is often difficult to say whether these unpublished reports represent interim data and analysis or completed trials. This notwithstanding, the two relatively small surfactant comparison studies available only in abstract form and missing from this review affected just the comparison of Survanta with Exosurf; not including them in the calculations did not change the results of the meta-analysis. In this review, the authors establish the relative quality of the available studies using a known evaluation scale [15]. Recognizing that many instruments for quality assessment of clinical trials are available, this choice was based on the fact that this scale has been extensively used and validated, and it pays particular attention to issues of study design and reporting aimed at minimizing biases. The assessment score considers randomization, blinding, and reporting of withdrawals to assess the quality of clinical trials. Considerable importance within the score is given to blinding because of the fact that there is compelling evidence to demonstrate that unmasked studies are more prone to bias [15]. Moreover, blinding acquires more relevance when physician-driven outcomes are used.

In this review, all calculations were done applying a random effects model, which assumes that the included studies are a random sample of a population of studies addressing the question posed. It is important to highlight the fact that several contemporaneous trials have appropriately used logistic regression to adjust some of the results by known confounders, such as the effect of center (in a multicenter study), birth weight or gestational age stratification, and other variables. The calculations for this review were generated using RevMan 4.2 (Information Management Systems, Copenhagen, Denmark)—used in The Cochrane Collaboration—in which the input consists of unadjusted raw data; therefore, the results reported may not be similar to those of the original publications. Finally, whereas there are many outcomes reported in surfactant comparison trials, the authors have focused primarily on mortality, given its importance and obvious ease and consistency of definition. Other important outcomes that are focused on, such as BPD or chronic lung disease (CLD) and pneumothorax, can be ascertained with less reliability than mortality, or their diagnostic criteria have evolved. Nevertheless, they are important to clinicians and have been included in this review. If side effects during administration were evaluated, this has also been included. Decisions to choose one surfactant over another may be partially based on some of these minor issues. Therefore, having information about them from randomized trials, especially if appropriately masked, is far more important than that available in biased commercial brochures or personal experiences.

Head-to-head comparisons

Collectively, surfactant comparison trials represent data from many thousands of neonates (Table 2), although not all trials are of the same methodologic quality (Table 3). Most infants randomized in these trials

Table 2
Number of neonates enrolled in published surfactant comparison studies

Surfactant	Number randomized	Number in final analysis	% randomized in final analysis
Survanta	7406	7141	96.4
Exosurf	5813	5676	97.6
Infasurf	5277	5011	94.9
Surfaxin	1546	1537	99.4
Curosurf	1265	1222	96.6
Alveofact	331	331	100

Table 3
Quality assessment of clinical trials comparing different surfactants

Study	Randomization	Blinding	Withdrawals	Intention to treat	Score[a]
Ainsworth et al, 2000 [14]	Yes	No	13 patients	Yes	3
Attar et al, 2004 [20]	Yes	No	No	Not stated	2
Baroutis et al, 2003 [22]	Yes	Not stated	Not stated	Not stated	1
Bloom et al, 1997 [19]	Yes	Yes	54 patients	No	5
Bloom and Clark, 2005 [21]	Yes	Yes	No	Yes	5
Da Costa et al, 1999 [10]	Yes	No	No	Yes	2
Hammoud et al, 2004 [23]	Yes	Incomplete	No	Yes	3
Horbar et al, 1993 [6]	Yes	No	3 patients	Yes	2
Hudak et al, 1996 [11]	Yes	Yes	100 patients	No	5
Hudak et al, 1997 [12]	Yes	Yes	25 patients	No	5
Kukkonen et al, 2000 [13]	Yes	No	7 patients	Yes	2
Malloy et al, 2005 [27]	Yes	Not stated	2 patients	Not stated	2
Modanlou et al, 1997 [9]	Yes	No	No	Yes	1
Moya et al, 2005 [16]	Yes	Yes	No	Yes	5
Ramanathan et al, 2004 [26]	Yes	Incomplete	8 patients	No	4
Sehgal et al, 1994 [7]	Yes	No	1 patient	Yes	3
Sinha et al, 2005 [32]	Yes	Adequate	9 patients	No	4
Speer et al, 1995 [25]	Yes	No	2 patients	Yes	2
Vermont-Oxford Neonatal Network, 1996 [8]	Yes	No	No	Yes	2
Yalaz et al, 2004 [24]	Yes	Not stated	No	Not stated	2

[a] *Data from* Jadad AR, Moore RA, Carroll D, et al. Assessing the quality of reports of randomized clinical trials: is blinding necessary? Control Clin Trials 1996;17:1–12.

have been part of the final results, connoting a commitment to conduct intention-to-treat analyses. The use of surfactant has evolved since the first trials comparing surfactant with placebo were published. Current practice includes prophylactic or early administration of surfactant primarily to infants who weigh less than 1000 g or are less than 28 to 29 weeks of age, and, in general, overall earlier administration of rescue surfactant to infants with established RDS. Also, many neonatal intensive care units (NICUs)

Table 4
Main characteristics of surfactant comparison studies

Comparison	Total N R (A)	Subjects	Approach	Antenatal steroids	Primary outcome(s)
Survanta versus Exosurf					
Horbar et al, 1993 [6]	614 (614)	501–1500 g	Treatment	17%	Death or BPD at 28 days and Fio_2 plus MAP
Seghal et al, 1994 [7]	41 (40)	600–1750 g	Treatment	Not reported	Ventilatory measures
Vermont-Oxford Neonatal Network, 1996 [8]	1296 (1296)	501–1500 g	Treatment	33%	Death or CLD at 28 days
Modanlou et al, 1997 [9]	122 (122)	500–1500 g	Treatment	43%	Unknown
Da Costa et al, [10]	89 (89)	>999 g and <37 weeks	Treatment	36%	Death or CLD at 28 days and OI at 24 hours
Moya et al, 2005 [16]	767 (767)	600–1250 g and <32 weeks	Prophylaxis	76%	RDS at 24 hours and RDS-related deaths
Survanta versus Infasurf					
Bloom et al, 1997 [19]					
Treatment	662 (608)	≤2000 g	Treatment	10%	25% reduction, third dose surfactant
Prevention	457 (374)	≤1250 g	Prevention	27%	25% reduction, second dose surfactant
Attar et al, 2004 [20]	40 (40)	<37 weeks	Treatment	82%	Pulmonary compliance after first dose
Bloom and Clark, 2005 [21]					
Treatment	1361 (1361)	401–2000 g	Treatment	73%	Survival without BPD (36 weeks)
Prevention	749 (749)	23 to <30 weeks	Prevention	91%	Survival without BPD (36 weeks)
Survanta versus Alveofact					
Baroutis et al, 2003 [22]	53 (53)	<32 weeks and <2000 g	Treatment	32%	Unspecified
Hammoud et al, 2004 [23]	109 (109)	<34 weeks	Treatment	71%	CLD at 28 days
Yalaz et al, 2004 [24]	50 (50)	<36 weeks	Treatment	66%	Unspecified
Curosurf versus Survanta					
Speer et al, 1995 [25]	75 (73)	700–1500 g	Treatment	40%	Unspecified
Baroutis et al, 2003 [22]	53 (53)	<32 weeks and <2000 g	Treatment	28%	Unspecified

Study	A (analyzed)	GA/BW	Mode	%	Outcome
Ramanathan et al, 2004 [26]	301 (293)	<35 weeks and 750–1750 g	Treatment	81%	Integrated Fio₂ requirement 6 hours after first dose
Malloy et al, 2005 [27]	60 (58)	<37 weeks	Treatment	74%	Fio₂ requirement 48 hours after first dose surfactant
Curosurf versus Exosurf					
Kukkonen et al, 2000 [13]	235 (228)	No limit GA/BW	Treatment	59%	Duration MV, duration O₂ >30%
Murdoch and Kempley, 2000 [28]	24 (22)	25–36 weeks	Treatment	Not reported	Effect on blood flows
Curosurf versus Pumactant					
Ainsworth et al, 2000 [14]	212 (199)	25 to <30 weeks	Treatment	93%	Days spent in intensive care
Infasurf versus Exosurf					
Hudak et al, 1996 [11]	1133 (1033)	No limit GA/BW	Treatment	Not reported	Air leak before 7 days, RDS-related deaths, survival without BPD (28 days), mean Fio₂ and MAP first 72 hours
Hudak et al, 1997 [12]	871 (846)	<29 weeks	Prophylaxis	33%	RDS, RDS-related deaths, survival without BPD (28 days)
Surfaxin versus Exosurf					
Moya et al, 2005 [16]	1036 (1036)	24–32 weeks and 600–1250 g	Prophylaxis	78%	RDS, death related to RDS first 14 days
Surfaxin versus Survanta					
Moya et al, 2005 [16]	785 (785)	24–32 weeks and 600–1250 g	Prophylaxis	77%	RDS, death related to RDS first 14 days
Surfaxin versus Curosurf					
Sinha et al, 2005 [32]	252 (243)	24–28 weeks and 600–1250 g	Prophylaxis	86%	Survival without BPD (28 days)

Abbreviations: A, analyzed; BDP, bronchopulmonary dysplasia; BW, body weight; CLD, chronic lung disease; Fio₂, fraction of inspired oxygen; GA, gestational age; MAP, mean arterial pressure; MV, mechanical ventilation; OI, oxygenation index; R, randomized; RDS, respiratory distress syndrome.

use early continuous positive airway pressure (CPAP), with or without surfactant administration, and various modalities of patient-triggered ventilation. In addition, there has been a marked increase in the use of antenatal steroids reported in surfactant comparison trials published after the mid-1990s (Table 4).

Survanta versus other surfactants

Survanta has been compared with Exosurf (six published trials), Infasurf (three published trials), and Alveofact (two smaller trials). The quality assessment and main characteristics of these trials are shown in Tables 3 and 4. Survanta has also been compared with Curosurf in four published trials and with Surfaxin in one study.

Survanta versus Exosurf

All studies comparing Survanta with Exosurf were for treatment of RDS with the exception of the recent Surfaxin prophylaxis trial comparing Surfaxin with Exosurf, in which infants were also randomized to Survanta in a 2:2:1 scheme [16]. None of these trials were masked, except for the comparison nested within the Surfaxin trial. Given the potential for different results, in the authors' review, the comparisons of Survanta with Exosurf were made separately for treatment and prophylaxis trials (Table 5). A brief description of the trials that compared these surfactants is found in the following sections.

Horbar and colleagues, 1993

This multicenter study was not masked but was analyzed on an intention-to-treat basis [6]. Its quality assessment is affected primarily by the lack of blinding. It was conducted between 1991 and 1992 and enrolled 614 infants with an average birth weight of 925 g and average gestational age of 26.8 weeks. The use of antenatal steroids was only 17% in both groups. Both surfactants were given as recommended by the manufacturers, and side effects during administration were recorded. There were no stated guidelines to determine changes in ventilatory support and fraction of inspired oxygen (Fio_2). Death before discharge was reported, and the diagnosis of BPD was established clinically and radiographically at 28 days, although oxygen use at 36 weeks–corrected age was also reported. Infants received either surfactant at an average of 4.5 hours while on an average Fio_2 of 0.75 with a mean airway pressure (Paw) of 10 cm H_2O. There was a significant difference in the initial response favoring Survanta but no significant differences in any neonatal morbidity or duration of ventilation or supplemental oxygen. Side effects during administration occurred in between 12% and 70% of infants, with some differences between surfactants.

Table 5
Survanta versus Exosurf for treatment or prophylaxis of respiratory distress syndrome

Study	Survanta	Exosurf	RR (95% CI)	Total N
Treatment of RDS				
Mortality before discharge				
Horbar et al, 1993 [6]	70/306	81/308	0.87 (0.66–1.15)	614
Sehgal et al, 1994 [7]	6/19	8/21	0.83 (0.35–1.95)	40
Vermont-Oxford Neonatal Network, 1996 [8]	108/652	121/644	0.88 (0.70–1.12)	1296
Modanlou et al, 1997 [9]	15/61	12/61	1.25 (0.64–2.45)	122
da Costa et al, 1999 [10]	1/46	4/43	0.23 (0.03–2.01)	89
Total	200/1084	226/1077	0.89 (0.75–1.05)	2161
Oxygen requirement at 36 weeks–corrected age				
Horbar et al, 1993 [6]	72/306	75/308	0.97 (0.73–1.28)	614
Vermont-Oxford Neonatal Network, 1996 [8]	153/652	169/644	0.89 (0.74–1.08)	1296
Total	225/958	244/952	0.92 (0.78–1.07)	1910
Pneumothorax				
Horbar et al, 1993 [6]	27/306	39/308	0.70 (0.44–1.11)	614
Vermont-Oxford Neonatal Network, 1996 [8]	153/652	169/644	0.60 (0.44–0.81)	1295
Modanlou et al, 1997 [9]	1/61	4/61	0.25 (0.03–2.17)	122
da Costa et al, 1999 [10]	1/46	5/43	0.19 (0.02–1.54)	89
Total	87/1064	144/1056	0.61 (0.47–0.78)	2120
Prophylaxis of RDS				
Mortality before discharge				
Moya et al, 2005 [16]	68/258	121/509	1.11 (0.86–1.43)	767
Total	68/258	121/509	1.11 (0.86–1.43)	767
Oxygen requirement at 36 weeks–corrected age				
Moya et al, 2005 [16]	109/258	229/509	0.94 (0.79–1.12)	767
Total	109/258	229/509	0.94 (0.79–1.12)	767
Pneumothorax				
Moya et al, 2005 [16]	14/258	35/509	0.79 (0.43–1.44)	767
Total	14/258	35/509	0.79 (0.43–1.44)	767

Abbreviations: CI, confidence interval; RDS, respiratory distress syndrome; RR, relative risk.

Sehgal and colleagues, 1994

This small single-center study was not masked and was conducted between 1989 and 1990 [7]. It randomized 41 infants, of whom 40 were analyzed. They had birth weights between 935 and 1075 g and an average gestational age of 28 to 29 weeks. The use of antenatal steroids was not reported. In general, both surfactants were given as recommended by the manufacturers, but side effects during administration were not recorded. There were no stated guidelines to determine changes in ventilatory support and Fio_2. Overall deaths were reported, but the timing of these was not stated (eg, at discharge). The diagnosis of BPD was established clinically and radiographically at 28 days, but the proportion of infants in oxygen at 36 weeks–corrected age was not reported. The timing of initial surfactant administration was not described, but it seems that infants had an oxygenation index (OI) of 13 to 16 and had, on average, a mean Paw of 9 to 10 cm H_2O just before administration of surfactant. There was a more significant improvement in ventilatory measures favoring Survanta but no significant differences in neonatal morbidity or mortality.

Vermont-Oxford Neonatal Network, 1996

This large multicenter study was not masked but was analyzed on an intention-to-treat basis [8]. Like the trial conducted by Horbar and colleagues [6], its quality assessment was primarily lowered by the lack of blinding. It was conducted between 1992 and 1993 and enrolled 1296 infants with an average birth weight of 985 g and average gestational age of 27.4 weeks. The use of antenatal steroids was only 32% to 34% in both groups. Both surfactants were given as recommended by the manufacturers, but side effects during administration were not recorded. There were no stated guidelines to determine changes in ventilatory support and Fio_2. Death before discharge was reported, and the diagnosis of CLD was established clinically and radiographically at 28 days, although oxygen use at 36 weeks–corrected age was also reported. Infants received either surfactant at an average of 3.0 hours while on an average Fio_2 of 0.73 to 0.75 with a mean Paw of 9.5 cm H_2O. There was a more rapid decrease of Fio_2 and ventilatory support favoring Survanta. There was no significant difference in the primary outcome of death or CLD at 28 days in the overall population, except for a lower incidence in the subset of infants weighing between 1001 and 1500 g treated with Survanta. The occurrence of pneumothorax was significantly lower in the Survanta group, but other neonatal morbidities were no different.

Modanlou and colleagues, 1997

This was a single-center unmasked study conducted between 1990 and 1993 [9]. The report also includes nonrandomized infants, but these were analyzed separately. The analysis for the 122 infants randomized was done on an intention-to-treat basis. They had birth weights between 950 and 970 g and an average gestational age of 27 weeks. The use of antenatal steroids ranged from 33% to 39%. In general, both surfactants were given as recommended by the manufacturers, but side effects during administration were not recorded. There were no stated guidelines to determine changes in ventilatory support and Fio_2. Overall deaths were reported, but the timing of these was not stated (eg, at discharge). The diagnosis of BPD was established clinically and radiographically at 28 days, but the proportion of infants in oxygen at 36 weeks–corrected age was not reported. Initial surfactant administration occurred around 6 hours after delivery while infants were on an average Fio_2 of 0.77 with an average mean Paw of 8 cm H_2O. As demonstrated in other trials, more rapid weaning was observed among infants treated with Survanta, but there were no differences in overall mortality or other complications, including pneumothorax.

da Costa and colleagues, 1999

This was a single-center unmasked study conducted between 1993 and 1996 [10]. All 89 infants randomized were analyzed on an intention-to-treat basis. They had median birth weights between 1300 and 1370 g and an average gestational age of 29 to 30 weeks. The use of antenatal steroids was between 32% and 39%. Both surfactants were given initially as recommended by the manufacturers, but subsequent doses were not given if there was no apparent response to the first dose (decrease in Fio_2 by 0.3). Side effects during administration were not recorded. There were stated guidelines to determine changes in ventilatory support and Fio_2. Overall deaths were reported, and all occurred before 28 days. The diagnosis of CLD was established clinically at 28 days, but the proportion of infants in oxygen at 36 weeks–corrected age was not reported. The timing of initial surfactant administration was not reported, but infants seemed to be on an average OI of 22 to 23 before surfactant was given. Faster weaning was observed among infants treated with Survanta, but there were no differences in overall mortality or other neonatal complications, including pneumothorax.

Data from these trials singly or in aggregate demonstrate no survival advantage for Survanta over Exosurf (see Table 5). Furthermore, no benefits in terms of the need for oxygen at 36 weeks–corrected age have been reported in any of these trials or were seen in the cumulative analysis. An important reduction in the risk of pneumothorax and faster weaning were consistently reported in most trials and in the cumulative analysis. Data from the Surfaxin trial represent the only available comparison of prophylactic use of Survanta and Exosurf [16]. Although faster weaning favoring Survanta-treated infants was also reported, there were no significant differences in the major outcomes of interest for the authors' review. Collectively, these data suggest that the advantage of Survanta over Exosurf is not in major outcomes, such as mortality or BPD, but is rather reflected in faster weaning, which is in keeping with studies in vitro and in animal models of RDS, in which surfactants with surfactant proteins work more rapidly

[17,18]. Also, there are fewer pneumothoraces with Survanta when used for treatment but not prophylaxis of RDS, with a number needed to treat (NNT) of approximately 18 to prevent one pneumothorax.

Survanta versus Infasurf

The main difference between these two surfactants lies in their content of SP-B, which is higher in Infasurf (see Table 1). At the usual prescribed dose, both surfactants provide approximately the same amount of total phospholipids. There have been three controlled trials comparing these surfactants, two of which have included a large number of infants [19–21]. The characteristics and quality assessment of these trials are shown in Tables 3 and 4.

Bloom and colleagues, 1997

This large multicenter trial was conducted between 1992 and 1993 and included a prevention arm (infants <29 weeks of age with a birth weight <1250 g) and a treatment arm (infants weighing <2000 g with established RDS) [19]. It had a masked design, and sample size calculations were based on decreasing the need for repeat dosing of surfactant. Data published for the treatment arm reflected the evaluable population (92% of randomized infants), but the results were reportedly similar if an intention-to-treat approach was used for analysis. The treatment arm reported included 608 infants weighing approximately 1160 g and aged 29.2 weeks of gestation at birth. A complete course of antenatal steroids was given to 9% to 12% of study participants. To maintain masking, both surfactants were given in similar volumes and intervals (this was slightly different than standard dosing of Infasurf). Side effects during administration were recorded. There were no stated guidelines to determine changes in ventilatory support and Fio_2. Mortality at discharge and the proportion of infants in oxygen at 36 weeks–corrected age were reported. Initial surfactant administration occurred, on average, at 6 to 7 hours after delivery while infants were on an average Fio_2 of 0.75 with an average mean Paw of approximately 9 cm H_2O. Faster weaning and a lesser need for additional doses were observed among infants treated with Infasurf, but there were no differences in overall mortality or other neonatal complications, including pneumothorax. Dosing complications were seen in approximately 25% of the infants and were evenly distributed among both surfactants. The prevention arm was conducted between 1992 and early 1994. Data published on the evaluable population of the prevention arm represent 82% of randomized infants, but the results were reportedly similar if an intention-to-treat approach was used for analysis. This arm included 374 infants weighing approximately 845 to 890 g and aged 27.1 weeks of gestation at birth. A complete course of antenatal steroids was given to 26% to 28% of study participants. Both surfactants were given as in the treatment arm. Side effects during administration were recorded. There were no stated guidelines to determine changes in ventilatory support and Fio_2. Mortality at discharge and the proportion of infants in oxygen at 36 weeks–corrected age were reported. Initial surfactant administration occurred within 15 minutes after delivery. Faster weaning among infants given Infasurf was not observed, but there was a shorter duration of supplemental oxygen and mechanical ventilation in this group. There were no differences in overall mortality or other neonatal complications, including pneumothorax (Table 6). Dosing complications were seen in fewer infants than in the treatment arm of the trial (18%), with no differences between surfactants.

Attar and colleagues, 2004

This small single-center treatment trial was not masked and used sample size calculations based on improvements in pulmonary dynamic compliance after surfactant administration [20]. Data were analyzed using an intention-to-treat approach. Only 40 infants weighing between 1300 and 1620 g and at 29 to 30 weeks of gestational age at birth were enrolled. Antenatal steroids were given to 79% to 86% of study participants. Both surfactants were given according to the manufacturers' recommendations. Side effects during administration were apparently not recorded. There were stated guidelines to determine changes in ventilatory support and Fio_2, and measurements of dynamic lung compliance were also used as criteria for retreatment with surfactant. Mortality at discharge and the proportion of infants in oxygen at 36 weeks–corrected age were reported. The timing of initial surfactant administration was not reported, but infants were on an average Fio_2 of 0.54 to 0.63 with an average mean Paw of approximately 8 to 10 cm H_2O before surfactant. Faster weaning and a lesser need for additional doses were observed among infants treated with Infasurf. Mortality was uncommon, and there were no pneumothoraces in either group. There were no differences between groups in any morbidity examined.

Bloom and Clark, 2005

This publication summarizes the outcomes of two trials relatively similar to those previously reported by these authors in 1997 but with a different scope and design [21]. As in the 1997 publication, there are prevention (23–29.6 weeks of gestation) and treatment (401–2000-g birth weight with RDS) trials within this report. These large multicenter trials were conducted between 2001 and 2003, and a decision to stop them prematurely was made because of slow enrollment. Both trials had a masked design, and sample size calculations were based on increasing survival to 36 weeks–corrected age without the need for supplemental oxygen and not on the softer outcome of repeat dosing used previously. In both trials, data were analyzed and the results reported using an intention-to-treat approach. Seventy three percent and 90% to 93% of study participants were exposed to antenatal steroids in the treatment and prevention studies, respectively. The treatment trial included 1361 infants weighing approximately 1100 g and aged 28 to 29

Table 6
Survanta versus Infasurf for treatment or prophylaxis of respiratory distress syndrome

Study	Survanta	Infasurf	RR (95% CI)	N
Treatment of RDS				
Mortality before discharge				
Bloom et al, 1997 [19]	51/305	54/303	0.94 (0.66–1.33)	608
Attar et al, 2004 [20]	2/21	0/19	4.55 (0.23–89.08)	40
Bloom and Clark, 2005 [21]	70/673	77/688	0.93 (0.68–1.26)	1361
Total	123/999	131/1010	0.94 (0.75–1.18)	2009
Oxygen requirement at 36 weeks–corrected age				
Bloom et al, 1997 [19]	174/305	158/303	1.09 (0.95–1.27)	608
Attar et al, 2004 [20]	14/21	11/19	1.15 (0.71–1.88)	40
Bloom and Clark, 2005 [21]	205/673	210/688	1.00 (0.85–1.17)	1361
Total	393/999	379/1010	1.05 (0.95–1.17)	2009
Pneumothorax				
Bloom et al, 1997 [19]	30/305	18/303	1.66 (0.94–2.91)	608
Attar et al, 2004 [20]	0/21	0/19	Not estimable	40
Bloom and Clark, 2005 [21]	56/673	40/688	1.43 (0.97–2.12)	1361
Total	86/999	58/1010	1.50 (1.09–2.07)	2009
Prophylaxis of RDS				
Mortality before discharge				
Bloom et al, 1997 [19]	15/194	25/180	0.56 (0.30–1.02)	374
Bloom and Clark, 2005 [21]	45/375	49/374	0.92 (0.63–1.34)	749
Total	60/569	74/554	0.76 (0.47–1.22)	1123
Oxygen requirement at 36 weeks–corrected age				
Bloom et al, 1997 [19]	45/194	35/180	1.19 (0.81–1.77)	374
Bloom and Clark, 2005 [21]	128/375	124/374	1.03 (0.84–1.26)	749
Total	173/569	159/554	1.06 (0.89–1.27)	1123
Pneumothorax				
Bloom and Clark, 2005 [21]	25/375	19/374	1.31 (0.74–2.34)	749
Total	25/375	19/374	1.31 (0.74–2.34)	749

In the report by Bloom and colleagues [19], only the proportion of infants with any air leak and not pneumothorax were reported.
Abbreviations: CI, confidence interval; RDS, respiratory distress syndrome; RR, relative risk.

weeks of gestation, whereas the prevention study enrolled 749 infants with a mean gestational age of 26.5 weeks and a mean birth weight of 900 g. Both surfactants were given as recommended by the manufacturers, and masking was maintained by having separate administrators. Side effects during administration were recorded. There were no stated guidelines to determine changes in ventilatory support and Fio_2 in either trial. Mortality at discharge and the proportion of infants in oxygen at 36 weeks–corrected age were reported. In the treatment study, initial surfactant administration occurred at a median time of 159 to 166 minutes after delivery while infants were on a median Fio_2 of almost 0.6. In the prevention study, infants received the first dose of surfactant at a median time of 8 to 9 minutes after delivery. Analysis of both trials after their premature closure and inclusion of more than 2000 infants did not reveal any differences in overall mortality or other neonatal complications, including pneumothorax. Dosing complications were reported in fewer infants than in their previous studies and were evenly distributed between both surfactants.

The cumulative analysis comparing Survanta and Infasurf did not reveal advantages favoring either surfactant in mortality at discharge or oxygen requirement at 36 weeks (see Table 6). There were significantly fewer pneumothoraces with Infasurf than Survanta when used for treatment but not for prophylaxis of RDS, with an absolute risk reduction of 2.9% (8.6% for Survanta and 5.7% for Infasurf) and an NNT of 35 infants (see Table 6). Also, in keeping with preclinical observations, there was evidence of a faster reduction of supplemental oxygen and ventilatory pressures with Infasurf than Survanta [18]. These findings suggest that a surfactant with more SP-B content but a relatively similar phospholipid composition may provide some short-term advantages, such as more rapid weaning and less pneumothorax, when used for treatment of RDS but does not reduce mortality or BPD.

Survanta versus Alveofact

The three trials comparing these two surfactants used only a treatment modality and included a relatively small number of subjects [22–24]. Some of them are of lesser methodologic quality than other surfactant comparisons (see Tables 3 and 4). Nevertheless, all infants entered in the three trials were analyzed. The recommended dose of Alveofact provides phospholipids at a rate of only approximately 50 mg/kg (in the standard volume of 1.2 mL/kg) compared with Survanta (100 mg/kg), but Alveofact has more SP-B than Survanta (see Table 1).

Baroutis and colleagues, 2003

In this single-center study, infants were randomized to receive Survanta (N = 26), Alveofact (N = 27), or Curosurf (N = 27) for treatment of RDS [22]. Only data for the Survanta-Alveofact comparison are discussed here. The trial was not masked, and sample size calculations were not reported. Although not clearly stated, it seems that data were analyzed using an intention-to-treat approach. Birth weights and gestational ages ranged between 1180 and 1230 g and 28 and 29 weeks, respectively. Antenatal steroids were given to less than 35% of study participants. Alveofact was given according to the manufacturer's recommendations; however, Survanta was slowly infused using a pump by means of a side port adaptor (this is a deviation from the manufacturer's recommendations and may have affected its distribution). Side effects during administration were apparently not recorded. There were some stated guidelines to determine changes in ventilatory support and Fio_2. Mortality at discharge, the proportion of infants in oxygen at 36 weeks–corrected age, and air leaks were reported, but pneumothorax was not a separate category. The timing of initial surfactant administration was not reported, but infants were on an average Fio_2 of 0.58 to 0.65 with an average mean Paw of approximately 8 cm H_2O before surfactant. There were no differences between groups in any major outcome examined, but the total duration of ventilation and oxygen therapy were marginally less in the Alveofact group (Table 7).

Hammoud and colleagues, 2004

This was a single-center randomized study for treatment of RDS [23]. The trial design included blinding of surfactant administration and sample size calculations. Data were analyzed using an intention-to-treat approach. Birth weights and gestational age ranged between 1030 and 1080 g and 28 and 29 weeks, respectively. Antenatal steroids were given to approximately 48% to 60% of study participants. Both surfactants were given according to the manufacturers' recommendations. Side effects during administration were not recorded. There were no stated guidelines for changes in ventilatory support and Fio_2. Mortality and pneumothorax were reported, but CLD was diagnosed at 28 days and not at 36 weeks–corrected age. Initial surfactant administration occurred at a median of approximately 2 hours in both groups while infants were on an average Fio_2 of 0.60 to 0.65 with an average mean Paw of approximately 9 cm H_2O. There were no advantages of either surfactant in mortality or pneumothorax, but days of ventilation and oxygen therapy were less in the Survanta group. Likewise, CLD at 28 days was less frequent among infants treated with Survanta.

Yalaz and colleagues, 2004

This single-center randomized study included 50 infants with established RDS [24]. The trial was unmasked, and sample size calculations were not provided. Data were reported on all randomized infants. Birth weights and gestational ages ranged between 1170 and 1250 g and 29 and 30 weeks, respectively. Antenatal steroids were given to 64% to 68% of study participants. Both surfactants were given according to each manufacturer's recommendations. Side effects during administration were not recorded. There were some stated guidelines for changes in ventilatory support and

Table 7
Survanta versus Alveofact in treatment of respiratory distress syndrome

Study	Survanta	Alveofact	RR (95% CI)	N
Mortality before discharge				
Baroutis et al, 2003 [22]	6/26	7/27	0.89 (0.34–2.30)	53
Hammoud et al, 2004 [23]	9/55	6/54	1.47 (0.56–3.86)	109
Yalaz et al, 2004 [24][a]	3/25	3/25	1.00 (0.22–4.49)	50
Total	18/106	16/106	1.12 (0.60–2.07)	212
Oxygen requirement at 36 weeks–corrected age				
Baroutis et al, 2003 [22]	4/26	3/27	1.38 (0.34–5.60)	53
Yalaz et al, 2004 [24]	1/25	1/25	1.00 (0.37–4.48)	50
Total	5/51	4/52	1.29 (0.37–4.48)	103
Pneumothorax				
Hammoud et al, 2004 [23]	5/55	10/54	0.49 (0.18–1.34)	109
Yalaz et al, 2004 [24]	3/25	7/25	0.43 (0.12–1.47)	50
Total	8/80	17/79	0.47 (0.21–1.01)	159

Abbreviations: CI, confidence interval; RR, relative risk.
[a] Mortality at 28 days.

Fio_2. Mortality up to 28 days, BPD diagnosed at 36 weeks–corrected age, and pneumothorax were reported. Initial surfactant administration occurred at an average of 88 to 97 minutes after birth while infants were on an average Fio_2 of 0.66 with an average mean Paw of approximately 8 to 9 cm H_2O. There were no differences in morbidity and mortality between the two groups.

Data from the cumulative analysis are shown in Table 7. Evidence from these three small randomized trials did not show any major difference favoring either of these surfactants when used for treatment of RDS.

Curosurf versus other surfactants

This porcine-derived surfactant has the highest concentration of phospholipids per unit volume of any commercially available surfactant (see Table 1). It has been extensively studied, mostly in Europe, although the comparison studies of Curosurf versus other surfactants have not included as many infants as those comparing other surfactants (see Table 2). It has been recommended to use initial doses of 100 or 200 mg/kg of phospholipids. Use of the higher dose of Curosurf not only provides more phospholipids than Survanta, but either dose also provides more SP-B. Thus, comparison studies were analyzed according to what initial dose of Curosurf was administered. Four trials have compared Curosurf with Survanta [22,25–27], two have compared Curosurf with Exosurf [13,28], and one trial each has compared Curosurf with Pumactant and Alveofact [14,22]. Their quality assessment and characteristics are found in Tables 3 and 4.

Curosurf versus Survanta

Some of the trials comparing these animal-derived products used different initial doses of phospholipids. Therefore, the summary comparison of these surfactants using similar initial doses of phospholipids contains data from two trials [22,26], and that comparing a higher initial dose of Curosurf versus the standard dose of Survanta includes data from three studies [25–27]. Accordingly, these results are given separately in Table 8.

Speer and colleagues, 1995

This small multicenter trial conducted between 1991 and 1992 in five German NICUs was designed as a pilot study to determine possible differences between treatment regimens [25]. Thus, sample size calculations were not provided. The trial was unmasked, and both surfactants were given according to the manufacturers' recommendations. The initial dose of Curosurf used was 200 mg/kg. Data were not reported in all randomized infants (two exclusions). The birth weights and gestational age were 1080 to 1095 g and 29 weeks, respectively. Antenatal steroids were given to 37% to 42% of study participants. Side effects during administration were not

Table 8
Curosurf versus Survanta in treatment of respiratory distress syndrome

Study	Curosurf	Survanta	RR (95% CI)	N
Using similar initial doses of phospholipids				
Mortality before discharge				
Baroutis et al, 2003 [22]	5/27	6/26	0.76 (0.20–2.87)	53
Ramanathan et al, 2004 [26][a]	9/96	10/98	0.91 (0.35–2.35)	194
Total	14/123	16/124	0.86 (0.40–1.85)	247
Oxygen requirement at 36 weeks–corrected age				
Baroutis et al, 2003 [22]	4/27	4/26	0.96 (0.21–4.30)	53
Ramanathan et al, 2004 [26][a]	30/96	33/98	0.90 (0.49–1.63)	194
Total	34/124	37/123	0.90 (0.52–1.58)	247
Pneumothorax				
Ramanathan et al, 2004 [26][a]	6/96	5/98	1.23 (0.39–3.88)	194
Total	6/96	5/98	1.23 (0.39–3.88)	194
Using Curosurf with a higher initial dose of phospholipids				
Mortality before discharge				
Speer et al, 1995 [25]	1/33	5/40	0.24 (0.03–1.97)	73
Ramanathan et al, 2004 [26][a]	3/99	10/98	0.30 (0.08–1.05)	197
Malloy et al, 2005 [27]	0/29	3/29	0.14 (0.01–2.65)	58
Total	4/161	18/167	0.26 (0.09–0.71)	328
Oxygen requirement at 36 weeks–corrected age				
Speer et al, 1995 [25]	4/33	4/40	1.24 (0.29–5.40)	73
Ramanathan et al, 2004 [26][a]	36/99	33/98	1.13 (0.63–2.02)	197
Malloy et al, 2005 [27]	10/29	10/29	1.00 (0.34–2.95)	58
Total	50/161	47/167	1.11 (0.68–1.81)	328
Pneumothorax				
Speer et al, 1995 [25]	2/33	5/40	0.48 (0.10–2.34)	73
Ramanathan et al, 2004 [26][a]	3/99	5/98	0.59 (0.15–2.42)	197
Malloy et al, 2005 [27]	2/29	1/29	2.00 (0.19–20.86)	58
Total	7/161	11/167	0.67 (0.26–1.76)	328

Abbreviations: CI, confidence interval; RR, relative risk.
[a] 32 weeks or less gestational age.

recorded. There were no stated guidelines for changes in ventilatory support and FiO_2. Mortality up to 28 days, BPD diagnosed at 36 weeks–corrected age, and pneumothorax were reported. Initial surfactant administration occurred at approximately 3 hours after birth while infants had a median FiO_2 of 0.9 with an average mean Paw of 9 cm H_2O. Infants who received Curosurf needed lower ventilatory pressures and FiO_2 primarily during the first 24 hours after treatment, but the overall duration of mechanical ventilation and supplemental oxygen did not differ. There was a nonsignificant trend toward lower mortality among Curosurf-treated infants. There were no significant differences in BPD at 36 weeks–corrected age or pneumothorax (see Table 8).

Baroutis and colleagues, 2003

This was a single-center study that randomized infants with RDS to receive Alveofact and similar initial doses of Curosurf or Survanta (phospholipids, 100 mg/kg) [22]. Some details of this study have been discussed previously in this review, and only pertinent data for the Curosurf-Survanta comparison are discussed here. The median birth weights and gestational age were 1135 to 1280 g and 29 weeks, respectively. Mortality at discharge, the proportion of infants in oxygen at 36 weeks–corrected age, and air leaks were reported, but pneumothorax was not a separate category. The timing of initial surfactant administration was not reported, but infants were on an average FiO_2 of 0.58 to 0.68 with an average mean Paw of 8 cm H_2O before surfactant. There were no differences in mortality or CLD, but the total duration of ventilation and oxygen therapy favored the Curosurf group.

Ramanathan and colleagues, 2004

This is the largest study comparing Curosurf with any other surfactant [26]. It randomized infants with RDS to receive Curosurf in initial doses of 100 or 200 mg/kg or Survanta. This 20-center trial, conducted during 2000 and 2001, was masked only for administration of the first dose of surfactant. Its primary outcome was the area under the curve for FiO_2 during the first 6 hours after initial surfactant administration. Sample size calculations were conducted accordingly, and the target of approximately 100 infants per group was attained. Eight infants were randomized but did not receive any surfactant and were not included in the final analysis. The mean birth weights and gestational age were 1150 to 1190 g and 29 weeks, respectively. Antenatal steroid exposure was identified in 76% to 85% of study participants. Both surfactants were given according to the manufacturers' recommendations. There were no stated guidelines for changes in ventilatory support and FiO_2, however, and side effects during administration were not recorded. Initial surfactant administration occurred at approximately 3 hours after birth while infants were on a mean FiO_2 between 0.60 and 0.65 with an apparently similar mean Paw between groups, but these values were not reported. Mortality as well as the need for oxygen at 36 weeks–corrected age was reported only for infants less than 32 weeks of age. Pneumothorax was reported for the overall population randomized, however. Among infants aged less than 32 weeks, there was a survival advantage at 36 weeks–corrected age favoring the group receiving the larger initial dose of Curosurf versus those who received Survanta. There were no differences in the proportion of infants in oxygen at 36 weeks–corrected age or in pneumothorax. Also, during the first 6 hours after surfactant treatment, those infants receiving both initial doses of Curosurf needed, on average, between 5% and 10% less oxygen than those treated with Survanta.

Malloy and colleagues, 2005

This single-center study randomized 60 infants with RDS to receive an initial dose of 200 mg/kg of Curosurf or standard doses of Survanta [27]. It seems as though the trial was not masked, and sample size calculations were conducted based on a primary outcome of Fio_2 needs during the first 48 hours after surfactant treatment. Data were analyzed after two exclusions. The mean birth weight and gestational age were 1400 g and 29.5 weeks, respectively. Antenatal steroids were given to 69% to 79% of study participants. Both surfactants were given according to the manufacturers' recommendations. Side effects during administration were not reported. There were stated guidelines to determine changes in ventilatory support and Fio_2. Overall mortality, BPD diagnosed at 36 weeks–corrected age, and pneumothorax were reported. The timing of initial surfactant administration and mean Paw before surfactant were not reported, but infants were on an average Fio_2 of 0.47 to 0.49 before surfactant treatment. There were no significant differences in mortality, BPD, or pneumothorax, but infants receiving Curosurf required less oxygen during the first 48 hours after the initiation of surfactant.

In the cumulative analysis, there is a significant survival advantage only with the higher dose of Curosurf versus Survanta for treatment of RDS (see Table 8). This finding is promising, despite the fact that there were no benefits in oxygen needs at 36 weeks–corrected age or pneumothorax among survivors. Using either dose of Curosurf seems to result in a more rapid reduction of Fio_2 compared with Survanta. Nevertheless, it should be noted that the overall quality of the trials in which these results are predicated is not as good as other comparisons; therefore, bias could be a plausible explanation. These results do not stand when all trials comparing these two surfactants are combined, independent of the initial dose of Curosurf used (relative risk [RR] = 0.58, 95% confidence interval [CI]: 0.32–1.05). In addition, Curosurf and Survanta have not been compared using a prophylactic approach, and the number of total and extremely premature infants enrolled in these published trials is relatively small compared with other surfactant comparisons (see Table 2). This notwithstanding, these data suggest that using higher initial doses of phospholipids and SP-B may lead to benefit in more important long-term outcomes.

Curosurf versus synthetic surfactants containing only phospholipids

Two trials have compared Curosurf versus Exosurf [13,29], and one has compared Curosurf with Pumactant [14]. The latter product was studied primarily in the United Kingdom and in a much smaller number of patients. The comparisons versus Exosurf were for treatment of RDS, whereas the study versus Pumactant involved prophylactic or early administration (most patients received surfactant by 60 minutes after birth).

Curosurf versus Exosurf

Kukkonen and colleagues, 2000

This is the third largest trial comparing Curosurf with another surfactant [13]. It was conducted during 1994 and 1995 in three NICUs in Finland. In an unmasked fashion, it compared Curosurf (100 mg/kg) versus standard doses of Exosurf for treatment of RDS. Sample size calculations were performed for the primary outcomes of duration of mechanical ventilation and supplemental oxygen. Although data were analyzed on an intention-to-treat basis, this was done after excluding seven patients. The mean birth weights and gestational age were 1255 to 1295 g and 29.5 weeks, respectively. Antenatal steroids were given to 52% to 66% of study participants (a significantly higher proportion in the Curosurf group). Both surfactants were given according to the manufacturers' recommendations. Side effects during administration were not reported. There were no stated guidelines to determine changes in ventilatory support and Fio_2. Overall mortality, BPD diagnosed at 36 weeks–corrected age, and pneumothorax were reported. The timing of initial surfactant administration was not reported, but infants were on an average Fio_2 of almost 0.80 with a mean Paw of 9 cm H_2O before surfactant treatment. There was crossover use of surfactants, mostly in the Exosurf group. There was no difference in mortality, pneumothorax, or CLD, but survival without CLD marginally favored the Exosurf group. Culture-proven sepsis occurred more often among infants treated with Curosurf. This group also had lower oxygen requirements during the first 6 hours after administration of surfactant than the Exosurf group.

Murdoch and Kempley, 2000

This was a small single-center trial comparing Curosurf (100 mg/kg) with Exosurf. It randomized 24 infants with RDS, but only 22 patients were finally analyzed [28]. The trial was not masked and was aimed at examining the effects of these surfactants in cerebral and intestinal blood flow; however, this publication reported only data on fluid balance. Only one death is described, but it is unclear in which group this occurred. Furthermore, there is no information on the doses of surfactant used or other common outcomes seen among infants with RDS. Therefore, this trial was not added to the analysis.

Curosurf versus Pumactant

Ainsworth and colleagues, 2000

This is the fourth largest trial comparing Curosurf with another surfactant and the only one that has compared these two surfactants [14]. It was conducted during 1998 and 1999 in 12 NICUs in the United Kingdom. This unmasked trial sought to compare the effect of similar doses of Curosurf and Pumactant (100 mg/kg) in infants aged 25 to 29 weeks of gestation who were intubated for presumed RDS. The primary outcome measure was the duration of high-dependency care (need for respiratory support and supplemental oxygen). Sample size calculations performed accordingly estimated a need to recruit 241 infants per group. The trial was stopped by the Data Safety and Monitoring Committee when only 212 infants had been randomized, however, because of an unexpected difference in mortality between groups. Data were analyzed and reported after 13 infants were excluded (total reported = 199 infants). The median birth weights and gestational age were approximately 945 to 1025 g and 28 weeks, respectively. Antenatal steroids were given to more than 90% of study participants. Curosurf was given according to the manufacturer's recommendations, but this is unclear for Pumactant. Side effects during administration were not reported. There were no stated guidelines to determine changes in ventilatory support and Fio_2. Overall mortality, CLD diagnosed at 36 weeks–corrected age, and pneumothorax (needing a chest drain, which is different than other definitions) were reported. Approximately two thirds of the infants received the initial surfactant dose within 30 minutes of delivery. There was no difference in the primary outcome measure. There was an almost 60% lower predischarge mortality rate in the group treated with Curosurf compared with those who received Pumactant (14% versus 31%), however. This large difference, not seen in any other trial comparing surfactants, was largely attributable, per the authors, to the higher than expected mortality among Pumactant-treated infants. The striking mortality results of this trial drive to statistical significance the comparison of overall mortality between synthetic and animal-derived surfactants in the systematic review of Soll and Blanco [5]. No differences in CLD among survivors at 36 weeks–corrected age, pneumothorax, or any other complication of prematurity were observed.

Results from these trials demonstrate that using Curosurf lowers mortality only against the synthetic surfactant, Pumactant, but that this cannot be generalized to Exosurf (Table 9). Furthermore, no advantages of using Curosurf at an initial dose of 100 mg/kg over a synthetic surfactant containing only phospholipids in other complications of prematurity, such as need for oxygen at 36 weeks–corrected age or pneumothorax, have been reported. A higher dose of Curosurf has not been tested against synthetic surfactants containing only phospholipids. Ironically, if one compared Curosurf versus the combined synthetic surfactants, there would be no survival advantage of Curosurf (RR = 0.84, 95% CI: 0.25–2.81).

Table 9
Comparison trials of Curosurf versus synthetic surfactants

Study	Curosurf	Exosurf	RR (95% CI)	N
Curosurf versus Exosurf in treatment of RDS				
Mortality before discharge Kukkonen et al, 2000 [13]	23/113	15/115	1.56 (0.86–2.83)	230
Total	23/113	15/115	1.56 (0.86–2.83)	230
Oxygen requirement at Kukkonen et al, 2000 [13]	38/113	31/115	1.25 (0.84–1.86)	230
36 weeks–corrected age				
Total	38/113	31/115	1.25 (0.84–1.86)	230
Pneumothorax Kukkonen et al, 2000 [13]	11/113	11/115	1.02 (0.46–2.25)	230
Total	11/113	11/115	1.02 (0.46–2.25)	230
Curosurf versus Pumactant in prophylaxis or treatment of RDS				
Mortality before discharge Ainsworth et al, 2000 [14]	14/99	31/100	0.46 (0.26–0.80)	199
Total	14/99	31/100	0.46 (0.26–0.80)	199
Oxygen requirement at Ainsworth et al, 2000 [14]	46/99	42/100	1.11 (0.81–1.51)	199
36 weeks–corrected age				
Total	46/99	42/100	1.11 (0.81–1.51)	199
Pneumothorax Ainsworth et al, 2000 [14]	11/99	22/100	0.51 (0.26–0.99)	199
Total	11/99	22/100	0.51 (0.26–0.99)	199

Abbreviations: CI, confidence interval; RDS, respiratory distress syndrome; RR, relative risk.

Other comparisons of animal-derived versus synthetic surfactants containing only phospholipids

Infasurf versus Exosurf for treatment or prophylaxis of respiratory distress syndrome

Hudak and colleagues, 1996

This well-designed, multicenter, masked study was conducted between 1991 and 1993 in 21 NICUs in the United States [11]. It had four primary outcomes of interest: air leaks before day 7, severity of RDS during the first 72 hours, incidence of death from RDS, and survival without BPD at 28 days. Sample size calculations were based on the expected incidence of air leak. It randomized 1133 infants with established RDS, but between 8% and 9% of the infants in each group were excluded from the primary analysis. The average birth weight was between 1570 and 1650 g, and the average gestational age was between 30.5 and 31.0 weeks (this was significantly greater in the Infasurf group). The use of antenatal steroids was not reported. Both surfactants were given as recommended by the manufacturers, and side effects during administration were recorded. Crossover use of surfactant was permitted. There were no stated guidelines to determine changes in ventilatory support and Fio_2. Death before discharge was reported, and the diagnosis of BPD was established clinically and radiographically at 28 days and at 36 weeks–corrected age. The latter was not clearly reported, however. The cause of death was assigned by the local principal investigator using study definitions. Infants received either surfactant at an average of 11 hours while on an average Fio_2 of 0.75 with a mean Paw of almost 10 cm H_2O. There was a significant difference in the initial response to surfactant favoring Infasurf-treated infants. Also, there were fewer pneumothoraces in this group. There were no significant differences in overall mortality or mortality from RDS, however. Although Infasurf-treated infants had fewer days of supplemental oxygen greater than 0.30 and fewer days on assisted ventilation, the incidence of BPD did not differ. Side effects during administration occurred in between 4% and 58% of infants, with some differences between surfactants (more desaturations with Exosurf for dose 1, but more desaturations, bradycardia, and airway obstruction with Infasurf in subsequent doses).

Hudak and colleagues, 1997

This multicenter trial of prophylaxis of RDS was conducted between 1991 and 1993 in 10 NICUs in the United States [12]. Its three primary outcomes were the incidence of RDS, death from RDS, and survival without BPD at 28 days. Sample size calculations were based on the expected incidence of RDS. It randomized 871 infants, but 3% were excluded from the primary analysis. The average birth weight was 900 g, and the average gestational age was 26.5 weeks. Antenatal steroid exposure occurred in approximately one third of the infants. Both surfactants were given in masked fashion as recommended by the manufacturers, and side effects during administration were recorded. Crossover use of surfactant was permitted only after three treatments of the assigned product. There were no stated guidelines to determine changes in ventilatory support and Fio_2. Death at 36 weeks–corrected age was reported, and the diagnosis of BPD was established clinically at 28 days and at 36 weeks–corrected age. The cause of death was assigned by the local principal investigator using study definitions. Almost all infants received either surfactant by 30 minutes of life. There was a significant reduction in the incidence of RDS and RDS-related deaths favoring infants who received Infasurf. Also, these infants were weaned faster than those who received Exosurf. There were no differences in overall mortality, incidence of BPD, or air leaks, however. The incidence of any IVH or severe IVH and periventricular leukomalacia (PVL) was higher among those who received Infasurf; however, this may have been influenced by the higher proportion of early deaths from RDS in the Exosurf group. Side effects occurred in between 2% and 70% of infants during the various dosings and were significantly more common among infants who received Infasurf.

These data indicate that using a surfactant that contains SP-B, like Infasurf, for treatment of RDS results in more rapid weaning and less pneumothorax but no advantages in major clinical outcomes compared with Exosurf (Table 10). When used for prophylaxis, Infasurf is more effective than Exosurf in reducing the likelihood and severity of RDS as well as associated deaths but does not have an impact on major clinical outcomes, such as overall mortality or BPD. Furthermore, the approximately 50% higher rate of severe IVH and PVL associated with the use of Infasurf versus Exosurf is of some concern, especially because no follow-up data from this trial have ever been published.

Surfactant comparison trials involving peptide-containing synthetic surfactants

Over the past several years, a new generation of synthetic surfactants containing peptides that mimic the action of SP-B or SP-C have evolved. These products have the obvious pharmaceutic advantage of being quite precise and consistent in their specific components as well as completely avoiding any potential or theoretic concerns related to administering animal-derived products. Two such surfactants, Surfaxin and Venticute, are currently undergoing clinical testing, although only the former has been studied in neonates. Surfaxin (lucinactant) contains phospholipids and the peptide KL_4, which is a series of repeats of lysine and leucine. This peptide was modeled by Cochrane and Revak [29] after the tail end of human SP-B. Several studies in vitro and in animal models of RDS have demonstrated its efficacy in increasing lung compliance and decreasing surface tension in

Table 10
Infasurf versus Exosurf for treatment or prophylaxis of respiratory distress syndrome

Study	Infasurf	Exosurf	RR (95% CI)	N
Treatment of RDS				
Mortality before discharge				
Hudak et al, 1996 [11]	52/525	61/508	0.82 (0.58–1.17)	1033
Total	52/525	61/508	0.82 (0.58–1.17)	1033
Oxygen requirement at 36 weeks–corrected age				
Hudak et al, 1996 [11]	25/525	20/508	1.26 (0.71–2.22)	1033
Total	25/525	20/508	1.26 (0.71–2.22)	1033
Pneumothorax				
Hudak et al, 1996 [11]	29/525	52/508	0.54 (0.35–0.84)	1033
Total	29/525	52/508	0.54 (0.35–0.84)	1033
Prophylaxis of RDS				
Mortality before discharge				
Hudak et al, 1997 [12]	64/423	73/423	0.88 (0.64–1.19)	846
Total	64/423	73/423	0.88 (0.64–1.19)	846
Oxygen requirement at 36 weeks–corrected age				
Hudak et al, 1997 [12]	50/423	41/423	1.22 (0.83–1.80)	846
Total	50/423	41/423	1.22 (0.83–1.80)	846
Pneumothorax				
Hudak et al, 1997 [12]	16/423	26/423	0.62 (0.34–1.13)	846
Total	16/423	26/423	0.62 (0.34–1.13)	846

Abbreviations: CI, confidence interval; RDS, respiratory distress syndrome; RR, relative risk.

a concentration-dependent manner [29,30]. Furthermore, preclinical studies also suggest that this surfactant may have an anti-inflammatory effect in the lung [31].

Surfaxin versus Exosurf

Moya and colleagues, 2005

This is one of the largest surfactant comparison trials conducted to date [16]. It sought to compare the prophylactic use (administered before 30 minutes of life) of Surfaxin versus Exosurf among infants weighing 600 to 1250 g and aged 24 to 32 weeks of gestation. The trial also included a reference arm of infants randomized to Survanta with a randomization scheme of 2:2:1. This international study was conducted between 2001 and 2003 in 50 NICUs and randomized 1294 infants, all of whom were analyzed using an intention-to-treat paradigm. Surfactant administration was masked (separate administrators), and sample size calculations were performed. The primary outcomes were the incidence of RDS at 24 hours and death from RDS through 14 days of age. Both of these outcomes as well as the occurrence of air leaks were adjudicated by an independent panel unaware of group assignment. All surfactants were given according to the manufacturers' recommendations, and Surfaxin was used at a dose of phospholipids, 175 mg/kg (5.8 mL/kg). Side effects during administration were recorded. Crossover use of surfactant was not permitted. There were stated guidelines to determine changes in ventilatory support and Fio$_2$. Death before discharge was reported, and the diagnosis of BPD was established clinically by the need for supplemental oxygen at 28 days and at 36 weeks–corrected age. The mean birth weight and gestational age of infants enrolled were 970 g and 28 weeks, respectively. Antenatal steroid exposure was reported in 74% to 79% of infants. The authors reported that there were significantly fewer cases of RDS at 24 hours and deaths from RDS among infants receiving Surfaxin compared with Exosurf. Also, BPD at 36 weeks–corrected age was significantly lower among Surfaxin-treated infants. No differences between the Surfaxin and Exosurf groups in overall mortality, pneumothorax, or other complications of prematurity were identified, however. The major outcomes of interest are shown in Table 11. These results were obtained after analysis using a different methodology than in the original report, which used logistic regression. Weaning of oxygen and ventilatory support was more rapid with Surfaxin than Exosurf. Side effects during administration occurred in between 7% and 27% of infants, and some of them were slightly more common among infants receiving Surfaxin than Exosurf.

Surfaxin versus Survanta

Moya and colleagues, 2005

This comparison is nested within the same trial described previously, although only half as many infants were randomized to receive Survanta

Table 11
Comparison trials of Surfaxin

Study	Surfaxin	Exosurf	RR (95% CI)	N
Surfaxin versus Exosurf in prophylaxis of RDS				
Mortality before discharge				
Moya et al, 2005 [16]	111/527	121/509	0.89 (0.71–1.11)	1036
Total	111/527	121/509	0.89 (0.71–1.11)	1036
Oxygen requirement at				
36 weeks–corrected age				
Moya et al, 2005 [16]	212/527	229/509	0.89 (0.78–1.03)	1036
Total	212/527	229/509	0.89 (0.78–1.03)	1036
Pneumothorax				
Moya et al, 2005 [16]	35/527	35/509	0.97 (0.61–1.52)	1036
Total	35/527	35/509	0.97 (0.61–1.52)	1036
Surfaxin versus Survanta in prophylaxis of RDS				
Mortality before discharge				
Moya et al, 2005 [16]	111/527	68/258	0.80 (0.61–1.04)	785
Total	111/527	68/258	0.80 (0.61–1.04)	785
Oxygen requirement at				
36 weeks–corrected age				
Moya et al, 2005 [16]	212/527	109/258	0.95 (0.80–1.14)	785
Total	212/527	109/258	0.95 (0.80–1.14)	785
Pneumothorax				
Moya et al, 2005 [16]	35/527	14/258	1.22 (0.67–2.23)	785
Total	35/527	14/258	1.22 (0.67–2.23)	785
Surfaxin versus Curosurf in prophylaxis of RDS				
Mortality before discharge				
Sinha et al, 2005 [32]	42/119	41/124	1.07 (0.75–1.51)	243
Total	42/119	41/124	1.07 (0.75–1.51)	243
Oxygen requirement at				
36 weeks–corrected age				
Sinha et al, 2005 [32]	42/119	37/124	1.18 (0.82–1.70)	243
Total	42/119	37/124	1.18 (0.82–1.70)	243

Abbreviations: CI, confidence interval; RDS, respiratory distress syndrome; RR, relative risk.

compared with the Surfaxin and Exosurf groups [16]. This trial provided the only data available to compare the prophylactic use of Survanta versus Exosurf. In the original report, there was no statistically significant difference in the occurrence of RDS between infants who received Surfaxin or Survanta at 24 hours, but there were significantly fewer deaths from RDS among those who received Surfaxin. Furthermore, there was a marginally significant lower mortality at 36 weeks–corrected age favoring infants in the Surfaxin group. No differences in pneumothorax, BPD, or other complications of prematurity between groups were reported. Results from this comparison using the methodology specified for this review are listed in Table 11. Side effects during administration and weaning from oxygen and ventilatory support were comparable between these two surfactants. Even though this was not the primary comparison of interest in this trial, these data suggest that use of Surfaxin for prophylaxis of RDS results in fewer deaths from RDS and perhaps lower overall mortality compared with Survanta. It is tempting to speculate that these potential advantages may reflect the higher amount of the SP-B mimic found in Surfaxin.

Surfaxin versus Curosurf

Sinha and colleagues, 2005

This trial compared the prophylactic use (administered before 30 minutes of life) of Surfaxin versus Curosurf among infants weighing 600 to 1250 g and aged 24 to 28 completed weeks of gestation [32]. The study was conducted between 2001 and 2003 in 22 NICUs of Europe and North America. It randomized 252 infants, but based on its noninferiority trial design, the primary analysis was done per protocol and not by intention-to-treat (9 infants were not analyzed). Surfactant administration was masked, and sample size calculations were performed. The trial was stopped early because of slow enrollment before the sample size could be reached. The primary outcome was the incidence of survival without BPD through 28 days as reported by the investigators (not by an independent panel). Both surfactants were given according to the manufacturers' recommendations at a similar dose of phospholipids (175 mg/kg; slightly less than the usual dose of Curosurf [200 mg/kg], because this initial dose was not approved in all participating countries). Side effects during administration were recorded. Crossover use of surfactant was not permitted. There were no stated guidelines to determine changes in ventilatory support and Fio_2. Death before discharge was reported, and the diagnosis of BPD was established clinically by the need for supplemental oxygen at 28 days and at 36 weeks–corrected age. The mean birth weight and gestational age of infants enrolled were 930 g and 27 weeks, respectively. Antenatal steroid exposure was reported in 84% to 88% of infants. Survival without BPD through 28 days occurred in 37.8% and 33.1% of infants receiving Surfaxin or Curosurf, respectively (P = not significant). There were no differences in overall mortality, need for supplemental oxygen at 36 weeks–corrected age, pneumothorax, or other complications of prematurity. Also, side effects during surfactant administration were comparable. Thus, there seem to be no major differences in those clinical outcomes examined so far between these two surfactants.

A summary of the Surfaxin trials suggests that this new-generation surfactant seems to have some advantages over previous synthetic surfactants containing only phospholipids, presumably from the SP mimic, and is at least as good as currently used animal-derived surfactants.

Summary

Synthetic surfactants that contain only phospholipids and animal-derived surfactants have been available to prevent and treat RDS for the past 2 decades. In this review, the authors have evaluated the evidence from comparison trials of the various surfactants and have placed special emphasis on assessing the quality of these studies. Furthermore, they focused mainly on ascertaining differences in important outcomes, such as mortality and BPD. None of the animal-derived surfactants (including Survanta, Infasurf, and Curosurf) have been shown to reduce the risk of mortality or BPD when compared with Exosurf. The advantages of these animal-derived surfactants over Exosurf are primarily faster weaning and a reduced risk of pneumothorax when used for treatment of RDS. Only Infasurf has been compared with Exosurf for prophylaxis of RDS and resulted in fewer air leaks, fewer infants developing RDS, and a lower rate of RDS-related deaths. This did not translate into improvements in overall mortality or in less BPD, however.

Whenever side effects of surfactant administration have been prospectively evaluated in comparison trials, there have been no major differences identified or side effects have been more common with administration of animal-derived surfactants than with Exosurf. Collectively, these data indicate that the presence of SP-B in animal-derived surfactants primarily affords advantages in short-term outcomes over synthetic surfactants that contain only phospholipids.

Comparisons of the animal-derived surfactants Survanta and Infasurf, which essentially differ mainly in their SP-B content, have not shown any advantages in mortality or BPD. There may be a survival advantage of using a high initial dose of Curosurf, which provides more phospholipids and SP-B, compared with Survanta, but no differences in other important outcomes have been observed. Caution must be exercised when interpreting these data, however, because they are derived from studies of lesser quality and with a lower number of infants than other surfactant comparisons.

A new synthetic surfactant, Surfaxin, that contains not only phospholipids but a peptide that functions like SP-B, has been clinically evaluated in neonates. Clinical trials comparing Surfaxin with synthetic surfactants that contain only phospholipids or with animal-derived surfactants have yielded promising results and strongly suggest that this new surfactant functions better clinically than previous synthetic surfactants and is at least as good as currently available animal-derived surfactants.

Unfortunately, all surfactant comparison trials have significant differences among them and also contain design flaws. The ideal surfactant comparison trial that could definitively answer which of the currently available products is better has not been conducted. Furthermore, there is a paucity of publications on the follow-up of infants participating in surfactant comparison trials. Future trials comparing surfactants should be appropriately sized, use meaningful primary outcomes, incorporate blinding and other measures to decrease potential biases, and include a long-term follow-up component.

References

[1] Jobe AH. Why surfactant works for respiratory distress syndrome. NeoReviews 2006;7(2): 95–106.

[2] Yost CC, Soll RF. Early versus delayed selective surfactant treatment for neonatal respiratory distress syndrome. Cochrane Database Syst Rev 2000;(2):CD001456.

[3] Soll RF, Morley CJ. Prophylactic versus selective use of surfactant in preventing morbidity and mortality in preterm infants. Cochrane Database Syst Rev 2001;(2):CD000510.

[4] Halliday HL. Recent clinical trials of surfactant treatment for neonates. Biol Neonate 2006; 89:323–9.

[5] Soll RF, Blanco F. Natural surfactant extract versus synthetic surfactant for neonatal respiratory distress syndrome. Cochrane Database Syst Rev 2001;(2):CD000144.

[6] Horbar JD, Wright LL, Soll RF, et al. A multicenter randomized trial comparing two surfactants for the treatment of neonatal respiratory distress syndrome. J Pediatr 1993;123: 757–66.

[7] Sehgal SS, Ewing CK, Richards T, et al. Modified bovine surfactant (Survanta) versus a protein-free surfactant (Exosurf) in the treatment of respiratory distress syndrome in preterm infants: a pilot study. J Natl Med Assoc 1994;86:46–52.

[8] Vermont-Oxford Neonatal Network. A multicenter, randomized trial comparing synthetic surfactant with modified bovine surfactant extract in the treatment of neonatal respiratory distress syndrome. Pediatrics 1996;97:1–6.

[9] Modanlou HD, Beharry K, Padilla G, et al. Comparative efficacy of Exosurf and Survanta surfactants on early clinical course of respiratory distress syndrome and complications of prematurity. J Perinatol 1997;17:455–60.

[10] da Costa DE, Pai MGK, Al Kusaiby SM. Comparative trial of artificial and natural surfactants in the treatment of respiratory distress syndrome of prematurity: experiences in a developing county. Pediatr Pulmonol 1999;27:312–7.

[11] Hudak ML, Farrell EE, Rosenberg AA, et al. A multicenter randomized, masked comparison trial of natural versus synthetic surfactant for the treatment of respiratory distress syndrome. J Pediatr 1996;128:396–406.

[12] Hudak ML, Martin DJ, Egan EA, et al. A multicenter randomized masked comparison trial of synthetic surfactant versus calf lung surfactant extract in the prevention of neonatal respiratory distress syndrome. Pediatrics 1997;100:39–50.

[13] Kukkonen AK, Virtanen M, Järvenpää A-L, et al. Randomized trial comparing natural and synthetic surfactant: increased infection rate after natural surfactant? Acta Paediatr 2000;89: 556–61.

[14] Ainsworth SB, Beresford MW, Milligan DWA, et al. Pumactant and poractant alfa for treatment of respiratory distress syndrome in neonates born at 25-29 weeks' gestation: a randomised trial. Lancet 2000;355:1387–92.

[15] Jadad AR, Moore RA, Carroll D, et al. Assessing the quality of reports of randomized clinical trials: is blinding necessary? Control Clin Trials 1996;17:1–12.

[16] Moya FR, Gadzinowski J, Bancalari E, et al. A multicenter, randomized, masked, comparison trial of lucinactant, colfosceril palmitate and beractant for the prevention of respiratory distress syndrome among very preterm infants. Pediatrics 2005;115:1018–29.

[17] Hall SB, Venkitaraman AR, Whitsett JA, et al. Importance of hydrophobic apoproteins as constituents of clinical exogenous surfactants. Am Rev Respir Dis 1992;145:24–30.

[18] Cummings JJ, Holm BA, Hudak ML, et al. A controlled clinical comparison of four different surfactant preparations in surfactant-deficient preterm lambs. Am Rev Respir Dis 1992;145:999–1004.

[19] Bloom BT, Kattwinkel J, Hall RT, et al. Comparison of Infasurf (calf lung surfactant extract) to Survanta (beractant) in the treatment and prevention of respiratory distress syndrome. Pediatrics 1997;100:31–8.

[20] Attar MA, Becker MA, Dechert RE, et al. Immediate changes in lung compliance following natural surfactant administration in premature infants with respiratory distress syndrome: a controlled trial. J Perinatol 2004;24:626–30.

[21] Bloom BT, Clark RH. Comparison of Infasurf (calfactant) and Survanta (beractant) in the prevention and treatment of respiratory distress syndrome. Pediatrics 2005;116:392–9.

[22] Baroutis G, Kaleyias J, Liarou T, et al. Comparison of three treatment regimens of natural surfactant preparations in neonatal respiratory distress syndrome. Eur J Pediatr 2003;162:476–80.

[23] Hammoud M, Al-Kazmi N, Alshemmiri M, et al. Randomized clinical trial comparing two natural surfactant preparations to treat respiratory distress syndrome. J Matern Fetal Neonatal Med 2004;15:167–75.

[24] Yalaz M, Arslanoglu S, Akisu M, et al. A comparison of efficacy between two natural exogenous surfactant preparations in premature infants with respiratory distress syndrome. Klin Pädiatr 2004;216:230–5.

[25] Speer CP, Gefeller O, Groneck P, et al. Randomised clinical trial of two treatment regimens of natural surfactant preparations in neonatal respiratory distress syndrome. Arch Dis Child 1995;72:F8–13.

[26] Ramanathan R, Rasmussen MR, Gerstmann DR, et al. A randomized, multicenter masked comparison trial of poractant alfa (Curosurf) versus beractant (Survanta) in the treatment of respiratory distress syndrome in preterm infants. Am J Perinatol 2004;21(3):109–19.

[27] Malloy CA, Nicoski P, Muraskas JK. A randomized trial comparing beractant and poractant treatment in neonatal respiratory distress syndrome. Acta Paediatr 2005;94:779–84.

[28] Murdoch E, Kempley ST. The effects of synthetic and natural surfactant on fluid balance in acute respiratory distress syndrome. Eur J Pediatr 2000;159:767–9.

[29] Cochrane CG, Revak SD. Pulmonary surfactant protein B (SP-B): structure-function relationships. Science. 1991;254:566–8.

[30] Revak SD, Merritt TA, Cochrane CG, et al. Efficacy of synthetic peptide-containing surfactant in the treatment of respiratory distress syndrome in preterm infant rhesus monkeys. Pediatr Res. 1996;39:715–24.

[31] Kinniry P, Pick J, Stephens S, et al. KL4-surfactant prevents hyperoxic and LPS-induced lung injury in mice. Pediatr Pulmonol. 2006;41:916–28.

[32] Sinha SK, Lacaze-Masmonteil T, Soler AV, et al. A multicenter, randomized, controlled trial of lucinactant versus poractant alfa among very premature infants at high risk for respiratory distress syndrome. Pediatrics 2005;115:1030–8.

Expanded Use of Surfactant Therapy in Newborns

Thierry Lacaze-Masmonteil, MD, PhD

*Department of Pediatrics, Stollery Children's Hospital, University of Alberta,
Edmonton, Alberta, Canada*

Pulmonary surfactant, a multicomponent complex of several phospholipids, neutral lipids, and specific proteins, is synthesized and secreted into alveolar spaces by type II epithelial cells [1–3]. The main functions of pulmonary surfactant are reducing the collapsing force in the alveolus, conferring mechanical stability to the alveoli, and maintaining the alveolar surface relatively free of liquid. Phospholipids are responsible primarily for the surface tension–lowering activity of surfactant, but other components present in animal-derived surfactants also play important roles [4,5]. In this respect, the contribution of low-molecular-weight surfactant proteins (SPs), SP-B and SP-C, to structural organization and functional durability is essential [5,6]. Tightly associated with phospholipids, the hydrophobic proteins SP-B and SP-C play a major role in enhancing the biophysical activity of phospholipids [6–9]. These proteins promote the rapid absorption of phospholipids at the air-liquid interface and account for the sustained low surface tension activity after dynamic compression.

Exogenous surfactants usually are classified into three families [10] (also see the article by Moya and Maturana elsewhere in this issue): (1) the mammalian or animal-derived surfactant preparations (so-called "natural surfactant"), which are purified and extracted with organic solvents from either lung minces or lung lavages—their phospholipid concentration is above 80%, and all contain the low-molecular hydrophobic proteins SP-B and SP-C; (2) the first generation of synthetic surfactant preparations ("artificial surfactant"), which are composed mainly of dipalmitoylphosphatidylcholine (DPPC) and are protein-free; and (3) the emerging second generation of synthetic surfactant–containing recombinant surfactant proteins or synthetic peptides whose spatial structure resembles the whole or part of SP-B or SP-C [10,11] (also see the article by Moya and Maturana elsewhere in this issue). A fourth category is

E-mail address: thierrylacaze@cha.ab.ca

0095-5108/07/$ - see front matter © 2007 Elsevier Inc. All rights reserved.
doi:10.1016/j.clp.2007.01.001   *perinatology.theclinics.com*

human surfactant derived from amniotic fluid obtained during elective cesarean section. Because of the inherent difficulties in collecting this material, it never has been practical on a widespread scale.

Evidence for the impressive efficacy of either prophylactic (treatment within the first minutes after birth, regardless of respiratory status) or rescue (treatment usually after 2 hours, when signs of respiratory failure are present) administration in the treatment of prematurity-related respiratory distress syndrome (RDS) come from overviews and meta-analysis of more than 40 trials, in which nearly 10,000 infants have been enrolled [12]. These meta-analyses demonstrate a consistent 40% reduction in the odds of neonatal death after surfactant treatment, either natural or synthetic and administered as either a prophylactic or rescue treatment. All types (animal-derived, protein-free synthetic, and peptide-containing synthetics) of surfactant and both treatment strategies also have resulted in a significant 30% to 50% reduction in the odds of pulmonary air leaks (interstitial emphysema and pneumothorax). Because the increase in survival is observed mainly among extremely premature infants, the incidence of bronchopulmonary dysplasia (defined as the persistence of supplemental oxygen requirements at 28 days of life or 36 weeks of postmenstrual age) has not been reduced dramatically despite the widespread use of surfactant. Elsewhere in this issue of *Clinics in Perinatology*, Moya and Maturana provide a comprehensive review of surfactant therapy for the prevention and treatment of RDS in preterm infants.

Surfactant deficiency secondary to lung immaturity is not the only mechanism accounting for the occurrence of acute respiratory failure in newborns [13,14]. Rare inherited disorders of surfactant homeostasis with mutations in the SP-B and SP-C genes can cause acute neonatal respiratory failure [15,16]. Qualitative or quantitative deficit of surfactant often is involved in the pathogenesis of various respiratory disorders in late preterm or term babies, including meconium aspiration syndrome (MAS), pneumonia/sepsis, and congenital diaphragmatic hernia (CDH). Preterm infants who have or do not have initial RDS also eventually may exhibit a secondary surfactant deficiency during the course of a chronic lung disease or after an acute episode of lung injury, such as pulmonary hemorrhage (PH) or pneumonia/sepsis. All these disorders may represent potential targets for surfactant therapy. Most of the experimental or clinical studies reported so far have been performed with animal-derived surfactants, mainly because SPs improve resistance of phospholipids to inactivation.

Meconium aspiration syndrome

Perinatal aspiration of meconium is a cause of potentially severe respiratory failure in near-term, term, or post-term infants. The incidence of MAS has decreased during the past 10 years. In Australia and New Zealand, approximately 4.3 babies per 10,000 live births were intubated and mechanically ventilated with the primary diagnosis of MAS between 1995 and 2002 [17]. The pathophysiologic mechanisms of hypoxemia in MAS include acute airway obstruction, chemical pneumonitis with release of vasoconstrictive and inflammatory mediators, persistent pulmonary hypertension of newborns who have right-to-left extrapulmonary shunting, and surfactant dysfunction or inactivation [18]. The hydrophobic chloroform-soluble fraction of meconium is the most potent inhibitor of surfactant function [19,20]. Surfactant is inhibited by meconium in vitro and in vivo in a dose-dependent fashion, and the inhibiting effect on surfactant function—measured in vitro with a pulsating bubble surfactometer—of small amount of meconium can be overcome by increasing the concentration of surfactant [21]. Synthetic surfactant preparations containing recombinant or analog peptides are more resistant to meconium in vitro than natural animal-derived surfactant [22]. In animal models of MAS, surfactant bolus administration is associated with an improvement in mechanical properties, gas exchange, lung inflammation, and histology [23–27]. Several groups report encouraging results in uncontrolled studies with natural surfactant administered to infants who have severe MAS [28–30]. Three randomized controlled trials confirm some benefits of the administration of several boluses of a natural surfactant in the treatment of MAS [31–34]. Although overall mortality was no different between the treatment group and the placebo group in each of these trials, the administration of several doses of a natural preparation was found to improve oxygenation in all three, to reduce the need for extracorporeal membrane oxygenation (ECMO) therapy in two [31–33], and to reduce the risk of pneumothorax in one [31].

In contrast to RDS treatment, where only one dose usually is sufficient to improve oxygenation dramatically and permit extubation, long-lasting improvement in oxygenation usually was seen only after at least the second bolus, supporting the need of repeated doses 6 hours apart to overcome ongoing surfactant inactivation in infants who have MAS [31,32,34]. The need to titrate the ongoing inhibiting activity of meconium may account for the improved compliance observed after continuous infusion of surfactant over 1 hour compared with bolus administration in a rabbit model of MAS [35]. In this respect, by removing meconium, inflammatory cells, edema fluid, and surfactant inhibitors from the alveolar space, bronchoalveolar lavage with dilute animal-derived or protein-containing artificial surfactant may be a promising approach for the treatment of severe MAS. Assessed in animal models of acute lung injury [36–41], this method also was evaluated in the treatment of severe MAS in an open and a small randomized controlled pilot study [42,43]. In the latter trial, 25 infants who had severe MAS were submitted to a series of bronchoalveolar lavages with dilute lucinactant. A trend toward a more rapid improvement in oxygenation and a shorter duration of mechanical ventilation was observed in the treated group. However, 20% of the subjects had the procedure halted because of hypoxemia or hypotension. Based on these results, two phase 3 clinical trials have been initiated in the United States and Australia to assess the efficacy and the safety of bronchoalveolar lavage with dilute lucinactant or beractant in severe MAS.

Several groups have investigated the potential benefit of the addition of polymyxin B or different polymers, such as dextran, hyaluronan, or poly-ethyleneglycol, to surfactant preparations in vitro or in animal models of MAS [44–49]. By increasing the resistance to inhibition, the polymers–surfactant combination significantly improved oxygenation or compliance compared with surfactant alone. Although promising results were obtained, further evaluations, including long-term safety, of these combinations in animal models are warranted before they can be tested in human newborns.

Although so far it has not been approved specifically for this disorder by any regulatory agency, surfactant therapy using bolus administration seems to be effective in the management of MAS. It reduces the need for ECMO. In the Australian and New Zealand cohort, surfactant was given in 30.8% of intubated babies who had MAS and, according to a recent survey performed in the United Kingdom, natural surfactant therapy is considered useful for MAS, with a majority of institutions preferring bolus to lavage administration [17,50]. The optimal method of administration (lavage or bolus), preparation (natural or peptide-containing synthetic preparation), dosing, and time in the course of the disease when surfactant should be given remain to be determined, however.

Respiratory distress syndrome in late-preterm babies

Most of the evidence for the benefit of surfactant comes from investigations performed in low or very low-birthweight babies. Although RDS is rare in late preterm infants (34–36 weeks' gestation), it remains a concern because this population represents 75% of all preterm babies. According to two large retrospective cohort studies, the incidence of any respiratory distress in babies born at 35 and 36 weeks is 7.3% and 8.3%, versus 0.6% and 2.9% in babies born between 37 and 42 weeks, respectively [51,52]. In another large area-based retrospective study of all babies born alive in a defined area in the north of England in 1988–1992, the incidence of babies ventilated for RDS was 130 per 10,000 live births in babies born between 34 and 36 weeks' gestation, compared with 9 per 10,000 in babies born at 37 or 38 weeks' gestation [53]. Respiratory distress is more likely to occur in late preterm or full-term infants delivered by cesarean section before the onset of spontaneous labor [54]. Lack of clearance of lung fluid, relative surfactant deficiency, and secondary inhibition of surfactant function are the major pathophysiologic mechanisms of respiratory distress in late preterm babies [54]. Likely because late-preterm infants have high survival and low morbidity rates, no study has evaluated specifically the benefit of surfactant treatment in this population.

Neonatal bacterial pneumonia

Neonatal pneumonia may affect surfactant functions by various mechanisms. Inactivation by plasma-derived proteins and blood components present in the alveolar spaces (hemoglobin, fibrinogen, and immunoglobulins), induction of bacterial secretion of phospholipases, and injury to the alveolar epithelium responsible for the synthesis and the secretion of surfactant all may play a role. Because chorioamnionitis is associated causally with a substantial proportion of premature births, surfactant inactivation and deficiency may coexist. Moreover, because some of the surfactant components may play a role in lung defenses against infection (eg, SP-A and SP-D), surfactant deficiency may worsen the infectious process. Indeed, early administration of a high dose of a natural surfactant (poractant alfa) in a rabbit model of pneumonia, alone or in association with a specific immunoglobulin against group B streptococcus (GBS), is shown to prevent intrapulmonary proliferation of GBS [55,56]. Animals infected with GBS or *Escherichia coli* had improved lung function and oxygenation after administration of poractant alfa compared with infected animals treated with placebo [57,58]. In a retrospective review of a large series of preterm and term infants who had respiratory failure associated with GBS sepsis, improved oxygenation and decreased ventilatory requirements were observed after administration of natural surfactant [59].There currently is insufficient evidence, however, that surfactant treatment improves the long-term outcome of septic newborns who have respiratory failure.

SP-A and SP-D, two complex glycoproteins present in pulmonary surfactant, play a major role in the innate lung defense barrier against pathogenic organisms [60,61]. SP-A is capable of stimulating the production of oxygen radicals by alveolar macrophages. This property, shared by SP-D, involves interactions between the protein and a specific receptor on the alveolar macrophage. SP-A also is shown to bind endotoxins, several viruses, and lipopolysaccharides of gram-negative bacteria, enhancing the uptake of these pathogens by the alveolar macrophage. Both proteins also modulate the production of cytokines by macrophages and neutrophils. Knockout mice models for each protein are established; the deficient animals exhibit normal respiratory behavior at birth but are more susceptible to infections [62,63]. The two proteins also regulate the functions of lymphocytes and play a beneficial role in the modulation of the inflammatory process occurring in various pathologic circumstances [64,65]. Neither of these proteins currently is a component of animal-derived surfactants used therapeutically. Whether or not SP-A– or SP-D–enhanced surfactants might be beneficial in the treatment of pulmonary inflammatory of infectious diseases is a tantalizing hypothesis that might be addressed by clinical trials in the future [64,65].

Pulmonary hemorrhage

PH or hemorrhagic pulmonary edema, either isolated or complicating the course of RDS or MAS, usually occurs during the first week of life [66]. Distinct from traumatic bleeding, PH represents the most severe form of pulmonary edema and can present as a sudden and life-threatening event with limited therapeutic options. Risk factors include extreme prematurity, intrauterine growth restriction, severe initial illness, patent ductus arteriosus, and administration of surfactant [67]. The exact role of exogenous surfactant in triggering PH remains uncertain and controversial [67,68]. Hemoglobin and plasma proteins, such as fibrinogen, abundantly present in alveolar spaces after PH, are powerful inhibitors of endogenous surfactant [69,70]. This process may be reversed by increasing the surfactant/inhibitor ratio in the alveolar spaces. The administration of an animal-derived surfactant in infants who have isolated or lung injury–associated PH is shown to improve the oxygenation index and lung compliance in two uncontrolled reports [71,72]. Improvements generally were immediate and long lasting. Although further investigations are warranted, treatment with exogenous surfactant may be a reasonable option in compromised infants who have severe PH.

Congenital diaphragmatic hernia

Several, but not all, studies of animal models of CDH suggest that lung immaturity with surfactant deficiency may be associated with pulmonary hypoplasia and pulmonary hypertension, the two hallmarks of CDH [73–75]. In the lamb model, prophylactic administration of surfactant improves oxygenation, lung compliance, and pulmonary perfusion [76,77]. Whether or not a relative qualitative or quantitative surfactant deficiency exists in the fetus who has CDH, data in newborns who have CDH do not support surfactant deficiency [78–80]. Whereas a few controlled and small-sized studies suggest modest clinical improvement after surfactant administration [81,82], the sole small, randomized trial (17 patients) published thus far does not show clinical benefit [83]. Additionally, retrospective analyses of a large series of treated patients fail to support any benefit for the use of surfactant therapy in term babies who have CDH [84,85].

Bronchopulmonary dysplasia

Expression of SP-A and hydrophobic SPs (SP-B and SP-C) is altered in animal models of chronic exposure to high concentration of oxygen [86–88]. In the baboon model of bronchopulmonary dysplasia, relative deficiency of SP-B accounts for lower lung volume, whereas low amounts of SP-A and SP-C are indicators of risk for infection in the evolution of chronic lung disease [89,90]. Surfactant function measured by the pulsating bubble surfactometer and contents of SP-A, SP-B, and SP-C are altered in mechanically ventilated very preterm babies who experience episodes of lung infection or deterioration [91]. A significant but transient improvement in oxygenation after administration of beractant is reported in a small sample of babies who had stable chronic lung disease and mechanical ventilation [92]. Whether or not intermittent repeated doses of surfactant during the course of chronic lung disease or specifically during episodes of respiratory decompensation improve pulmonary outcomes currently is under investigation [93].

Summary

Although there is no doubt that administration of exogenous surfactant to very preterm babies who have RDS is safe and efficacious, surfactant inactivation or deficiency plays a role in the pathophysiology of other pulmonary disorders affecting newborn infants. Preliminary data suggest that there may be a role for surfactant administration to babies who have MAS, pneumonia, and possibly bronchopulmonary dysplasia. Further investigation is necessary but seems warranted.

References

[1] Creuwels LA, van Golde LM, Haagsman HP. The pulmonary surfactant system: biochemical and clinical aspects. Lung 1997;175:1–39.
[2] Griese M. Pulmonary surfactant in health and human lung diseases: state of the art. Eur Respir J 1999;13:1455–76.
[3] Goerke J. Pulmonary surfactant: functions and molecular composition. Biochem Biophys Acta 1998;1408:79–89.
[4] Veldhuizen R, Nag K, Orgeis S, et al. The role of lipids in pulmonary surfactant. Biochem Biophys Acta 1998;1408:90–108.
[5] Johansson J, Curstedt T. Molecular structures and interactions of pulmonary surfactant components. Eur J Biochem 1997;244:675–93.
[6] Weaver TE, Conkright JJ. Function of surfactant proteins B and C. Annu Rev Physiol 2001; 63:555–78.
[7] Whitsett JA, Weaver TE. Hydrophobic surfactant proteins in lung function and disease. N Engl J Med 2002;347:2141–8.
[8] Hawgood S, Derrick M, Poulain F. Structure and properties of surfactant protein B. Biochem Biophys Acta 1998;1408:150–60.
[9] Johansson J. Structure and properties of surfactant protein C. Biophys Biochem Acta 1998; 1408:161–72.
[10] Ghodrat M. Lung surfactants. Am J Health Syst Pharm 2006;63:1504–21.
[11] Curstedt T, Johansson J. New synthetic surfactants—basic science. Biol Neonate 2005;87: 332–7.
[12] Halliday HL. History of surfactant from 1980. Biol Neonate 2005;87:317–22.
[13] Finer NN. Surfactant use for neonatal lung injury: beyond respiratory distress syndrome. Paediatr Respir Rev 2004;5S:S289–97.
[14] Lacaze-Masmonteil T. Exogenous surfactant therapy: newer developments. Semin Perinatol 2003;8:433–40.

[15] Whitsett JA, Wert SE, Trapnell BC. Genetic disorders influencing lung formation and function at birth. Hum Mol Genet 2004;13:R207–15.

[16] Whitsett JA. Genetic disorders of surfactant homeostasis. Paediatr Respir Rev 2006;7S: S240–2.

[17] Dargaville PA, Copnell B, for the Autralian and New Zealand Neonatal Network. The epidemiology of meconium aspiration syndrome: incidence, risk factors, therapies, and outcome. Pediatrics 2006;117:1712–21.

[18] Dargaville PA, Mills JF. Surfactant therapy for meconium aspiration syndrome. Drugs 2005;68:2569–91.

[19] Gunther A, Seeger W. Resistance to surfactant inactivation. In: Robertson B, Taeusch HW, editors. Surfactant therapy for lung disease. New York: Dekker; 1995. p. 269–92.

[20] Dargaville PA, South M, McDougall PN. Surfactant and surfactant inhibitor in meconium aspiration syndrome. J Pediatr 2001;138:113–5.

[21] Moses D, Holm BA, Spitale P, et al. Inhibition of pulmonary surfactant function by meconium. Am J Obstet Gynecol 1991;164:477–81.

[22] Herting E, Rauprich P, Sticntenoth G, et al. Resistance of different surfactant preparations to inactivation by meconium. Pediatr Res 2001;50:44–9.

[23] Sun B, Curstedt T, Song GW, et al. Surfactant improves lung function and morphology in newborns rabbits with meconium aspiration. Biol Neonate 1993;63:96–104.

[24] Sun B, Curstedt T, Robertson B. Surfactant inhibition in experimental meconium aspiration. Acta Paediatr 1993;82:182–9.

[25] Sun B, Hertling E, Curstedt T, et al. Exogenous surfactant improves lung compliance and oxygenation in adult rat with mecinium aspiration. J Appl Physiol 1994;77:1961–71.

[26] Hilgendorff A, Rawer D, Doerner M, et al. Synthetic and natural surfactant differentially modulate inflammation after meconium aspiration. Intensive Care Med 2003;29 2247–54.

[27] Hilgendorff A, Doerner M, Rawer D, et al. Effects of a recombinant surfactant protein-C-based surfactant on lung function and the pulmonary surfactant system in a model of meconium aspiration syndrome. Crit Care Med 2006;34:203–10.

[28] Auten RL, Notter RH, Kendig JW, et al. Surfactant treatment of full-term newborns with respiratory failure. Pediatrics 1991;87:101–7.

[29] Khammash H, Perlman M, Wojtulewicz J, et al. Surfactant therapy in full-term neonates with severe respiratory failure. Pediatrics 1993;92:135–9.

[30] Halliday HL, Speer CP, Robertson B, et al. Treatment of severe meconium aspiration syndrome with porcine surfactant. Eur J Pediatr 1996;155:1047–51.

[31] Findlay RD, Taeusch HW, Walther FJ. Surfactant replacement therapy for meconium aspiration syndrome. Pediatrics 1996;97:48–52.

[32] Lotze A, Mitchell BR, Bulas DI, et al. Multicenter study of surfactant (beractant) use in the treatment of term infants with severe respiratory failure. Survanta in Term Infants Study Group. J Pediatr 1998;132:40–7.

[33] Soll RF, Dargaville P. Surfactant for meconium aspiration syndrome in full term infants. Cochrane Database Syst Rev 2000;2:CD002054.

[34] Chinese Collaborative Study Group for Neonatal Respiratory Diseases. Treatment of severe meconium aspiration syndrome with porcine surfactant: a multicenter randomized controlled trial. Acta Paediatr 2005;94:896–902.

[35] Robinson TW, Roberts AM. Effects of exogenous surfactant on gas exchange and compliance in rabbits after meconium aspiration. Pediatr Pulmonol 2002;33:117–23.

[36] Parenka HS, Walsh WF, Stancombe BB. Surfactant lavage in a piglet model of meconium aspiration syndrome. Pediatr Res 1992;31:625–8.

[37] Meister JC, Balaraman V, Ku T, et al. Lavage administration of dilute recombinant surfactant in acute lung injury in piglets. Pediatr Res 2000;47:240–5.

[38] Ibara S, Ikenoue T, Murata Y, et al. Management of meconium aspiration syndrome by tracheobronchial lavage, replacement of surfactant TA. Acta Paediatr Jpn 1995;37:64–7.

[39] Lam BCC, Yeung CY, Fu KH, et al. Surfactant tracheobronchial lavage for the management of a rabbit model of meconium aspiration syndrome. Biol Neonate 2000;78:129–38.

[40] Cochrane CG, Revak SD, Merritt TA, et al. Bronchoalveolar lavage with KL4-surfactant in models of meconium aspiration syndrome. Pediatr Res 1998;44:705–15.

[41] Zhang E, Hiroma T, Sahashi T, et al. Airway lavage with exogenous surfactant in an animal model of meconium aspiration syndrome. Pediatr Int 2005;47:237–41.

[42] Lam BC, Yeung CY. Surfactant lavage for meconium aspiration syndrome: a pilot study. Pediatrics 1999;103:1014–8.

[43] Wiswell TE, Knight GR, Finer NN, et al. A multicenter, randomized, controlled trial comparing Surfaxin (Lucinactant) lavage with standard care for treatment of meconium aspiration syndrome. Pediatrics 2002;109:1081–7.

[44] Taeusch HW, Lu KW, Goerke J, et al. Nonionic polymers reverse inactivation of surfactant by meconium and other substances. Am J Respir Crit Care Med 1999;159:1391–5.

[45] Tashiro K, Kobayashi T, Robertson B. Dextran reduces surfactant inhibition by meconium. Acta Paediatr 2000;89:1439–45.

[46] Lu KW, Robertson B, Taeush HW. Dextran or polyethylene glycol added to Curosurf for treatment of meconium lung injury in rats. Biol Neonate 2005;88:46–53.

[47] Lu KW, Goerke J, Clements JA, et al. Hyaluronan reduces surfactant inhibition and improves rat lung function after meconium injury. Pediatr Res 2005;58:206–10.

[48] Ochs M, Schuttler M, Stichtenoth G, et al. Morphological alterations of exogenous surfactant inhibited by meconium can be prevented by dextran. Respir Res 2006;7:86.

[49] Stichtenoth G, Jung P, Walter G, et al. Polymyxin B/pulmonary surfactant mixtures have increased resistance to inactivation by meconium and reduce growth of gram-negative bacteria in vitro. Pediatr Res 2006;59:407–11.

[50] Greenough A, Pulikot A, Dimitriou G. Prevention and management of meconium aspiration syndrome—assessment of evidence based practice. Eur J Pediatr 2005;164:329–30.

[51] Rubaltelli FF, Bonafe L, Tangucci M, et al. Epidemiology of neonatal acute respiratory disorders: a multicenter study on incidence and fatality rates of neonatal acute respiratory disorders according to gestational age, maternal age, pregnancy complications and type of delivery. Italian Group of Neonatal Pneumology. Biol Neonate 1998;74:7–15.

[52] Escobar GJ, Clark RH, Greene JD. Short-term outcomes of infants born at 35 and 36 weeks gestation: we need to ask more questions. Semin Perinatol 2006;30:28–33.

[53] Madar J, Richmond S, Hey E. Surfactant-deficiency respiratory distress after elective delivery at "term". Acta Paediatr 1999;88:1244–8.

[54] Jain L, Eaton DC. Physiology of fetal lung fluid clearance and the effect of labor. Semin Perinatol 2006;30:28–33.

[55] Herting E, Jarstrand C, Rasool O, et al. Experimental neonatal group B streptococcal pneumonia: effect of a modified porcine surfactant on bacterial proliferation in ventilated near-term rabbits. Pediatr Res 1994;36:784–91.

[56] Hertling E, Gan XZ, Rauprich P, et al. Combined treatment with surfactant and specific immunoglobulin reduces bacterial proliferation in experimental neonatal group B Streptococcal pneumonia. Am J Respir Crit Care Med 1999;159:1862–7.

[57] Hertling E, Sun B, Jarstrang C, et al. Surfactant improves lung function and mitigates bacterial growth in immature ventilated rabbits with experimentally induced neonatal group B streptococcal pneumonia. Arch Dis Child 1997;76:F3–8.

[58] Song GW, Robertson B, Curstedt T, et al. Surfactant treatment in experimental Escherichia coli pneumonia. Acta Anaesthesiol Scand 1996;40:1154–60.

[59] Herting E, Geffeler O, Land M, et al. Surfactant tretment of neonates with respiratory failure and group B streptococcal infection. Members of the collaborative European Multicenter Study Group. Pediatrics 2000;106:957–64.

[60] Kishore U, Greenhough TJ, Waters P, et al. Surfactant proteins SP-A and SP-D: structure, function and receptor. Mol Immunol 2006;43:1293–315.

[61] Sano H, Kuroki Y. The lung collectins, SP-A and SP-D, modulated pulmonary innate immunity. Mol Immunol 2005;42:279–87.

[62] LeVine AM, Kurak KE, Wright JR, et al. Surfactant protein A binds group B Streptococcus enhancing phagocytosis and clearance from lungs of surfactant protein-A-deficient mice. Am J Respir Cell Mol Biol 1999;20:279–86.

[63] Levine AM, Whitsett JA, Gwozdz JA, et al. Distinct effects of surfactant protein A or D deficiency during bacterial infection on the lung. J Immunol 2000;165:3934–40.

[64] Hartl D, Griese M. Surfactant protein D in human lung diseases. Eur J Clin Invest 2006;36: 423–35.

[65] Kingma PS, Whitsett JA. In defense of the lung: surfactant protein A and surfactant protein D. Curr Opin Pharmacol 2006;6:277–83.

[66] Papworth S, Cartlidge PHT. Pulmonary haemorrhage. Current Paediatrics 2001;11:167–71.

[67] Raju TN, Langenberg P. Pulmonary haemorrhage and exogenous surfactant therapy: a meta-analysis. J Pediatr 1993;123:603–10.

[68] Braun KR, Davidson KM, Henry M, et al. Severe pulmonary hemorrhage in the premature infant: analysis of presurfacatnt and surfactant eras. Biol Neonate 1999;75:18–30.

[69] Holm BA, Notter RH. Effects of haemoglobin and cell membrane lipids on pulmonary surfactant activity. J Appl Physiol 1987;63:1434–42.

[70] Kobayashi T, Nitta K, Ganzuka M, et al. Inactivation of exogenous surfactant by pulmonary edema fluid. Pediatr Res 1991;29:353–6.

[71] Pandit PB, Dunn MS, Colucci EA. Surfactant therapy in neonates with respiratory deterioration due to pulmonary hemorrhage. Pediatrics 1995;95:32–6.

[72] Amizura T, Shimizu H, Niida Y, et al. Surfactant therapy in neonates with respiratory failure due to hemorrhagic pulmonary oedema. Eur J Pediatr 2003;162:697–702.

[73] Rottier R, Tibboel D. Fetal lung and diaphragm development in congenital diaphragmatic hernia. Semin Perinatol 2005;2:86–93.

[74] Mysore MR, Margraf LR, Jaramillo M, et al. Surfactant protein A is decreased in a rat model of congenital diaphragmatic hernia. Am J Respir Crit Care Med 1998;157:654–7.

[75] Van Tuyl M, Blommaart PE, Keijzer R, et al. Pulmonary surfactant protein A, B, C mRNA and protein expression in the nitrofen-induced congenital diaphragmatic hernia rat model. Pediatr Res 2003;54:641–52.

[76] Wilkox DT, Glick PL, Karamanoukian H, et al. Pathophysiology of congenital diaphragmatic hernia. Effect of exogenous surfactant therapy on gas exchange and lung mechanisms in the lamb congenital diaphragmatic hernia model. J Pediatr 1994;124:289–893.

[77] O'Toole SJ, Karamanoukian HL, Morin FC, et al. Surfactant decreases pulmonary vascular resistance and increases pulmonary blood flow in the fetal lamb model of congenital diaphragmatic hernia. J Pediatr Surg 1996;31:507–11.

[78] Moya FR, Thomas VL, Romaguera J, et al. Fetal lung maturation in congenital diaphragmatic hernia. Am J Obstet Gynecol 1995;173:1401–5.

[79] Ijsselstijn H, Zimmerman LJI, Bunt JEH, et al. Prospective evaluation of surfactant composition in bronchoalveolar lavage fluids with congenital diaphragmatic hernia and of age-matched controls. Crit Care Med 1998;26:573–80.

[80] Cogo PE, Zimmerman LKJ, Rosso F, et al. Surfactant synthesis and kinetics in infants with congenital diaphragmatic hernia. Am J Respir Crit Care Med 2002;166:154–8.

[81] Bae CW. Exogenous pulmonary surfactant replacement therapy in a neonate with pulmonary hypoplasia accompanying congenital diaphragmatic hernia: a case report. J Korean Med Sci 1996;11:265–70.

[82] Glick PL, Leach CL, Besner GE, et al. Pathophysiology of congenital diaphragmatic hernia: exogenous surfactant therapy for the high-risk neonate with CDH. J Pediatr Surg 1992;27: 866–9.

[83] Lotze A, Knight GR, Anderson KD, et al. Surfactant (Beractant) therapy for infants with congenital diaphragmatic hernia on ECMO: evidence of persistent surfactant deficiency. J Pediatr Surg 1994;29:407–12.

[84] Lally KP, Lally PA, Langham MR, et al. Surfactant does not improve survival rate in preterm infants with congenital diaphragmatic hernia. J Pediatr Surg 2004;39:829–33.

[85] Van Meurs K, and the Congenital Diaphragmatic Hernia Study Group. Is surfactant therapy beneficial in the treatment of the term newborn infant with congenital diaphragmatic hernia? J Pediatr 2004;145:312–6.

[86] Allred TF, Mercer RR, Thomas RF, et al. Brief 95% O2 exposure effects on surfactant protein and mRNA in rat alveolar and bronchiolar epithelium. Am J Physiol 1999;276: L999–1009.

[87] King RJ, Coalson JJ, deLemos RA, et al. Surfactant protein-A deficiency in a primate model of bronchopulmonary dysplasia. Am J Respir Crit Care Med 1995;151:1989–97.

[88] Savani RC, Godinez RI, Godinez MH, et al. Respiratory distress after intratracheal bleomycin: selective deficiency of surfactant proteins B and C. Am J Physiol Lung Cell Mol Physiol 2001;281:L685–96.

[89] Awasthi S, Coalson JJ, Yoder BA, et al. Deficiencies in lung surfactant protein A and D are associated with lung infection in very premature neonatal baboons. Am J Respir Crit Care Med 2001;163:389–97.

[90] Ballard PL, Gonzales LW, Godinez RI, et al. Surfactant composition and function in a primate model of infant chronic lung disease: effect of inhaled nitric oxide. Pediatr Res 2006;59: 157–63.

[91] Merrill JD, Ballard RA, Cnaan A, et al. Dysfunction of pulmonary surfactant in chronically ventilated premature infants. Pediatr Res 2004;56:918–26.

[92] Pandit PB, Dunn MS, Kelley EN, et al. Surfactant replacement in neonates with early chronic lung disease. Pediatrics 1995;95:851–4.

[93] U.S. National Institutes of Health. Pilot trial of surfactant therapy for preterm neonates 5–21 days old with respiratory decompensation. Available at: http://www.clinicaltrials.gov/ct/show/NCT00165074?order=1.

ELSEVIER
SAUNDERS

CLINICS IN
PERINATOLOGY

Clin Perinatol 34 (2007) 191–204

Evidence-Based Use of Adjunctive Therapies to Ventilation

Thomas E. Wiswell, MD[a,*], Win Tin, MD[b],
Kirsten Ohler, PharmD[c]

[a]Center for Neonatal Care, Florida Hospital Orlando, 2718 North Orange Avenue,
Suite B, Orlando, FL 32804, USA
[b]The James Cook University Hospital, Marton Road, Middlesbrough,
Cleveland TS4 3BW, UK
[c]Department of Pharmacy Practice, University of Illinois at Chicago,
833 S. Wood Street (M/C 886), Chicago, IL 60612, USA

Respiratory distress is the most common reason for admission to newborn intensive care units (NICUs). There is as wide a variation in the size and gestation of affected infants as there is in the types of respiratory disorders. Over the past two decades, we have witnessed a revolution in the therapies that are used to manage neonates who have pulmonary disorders, including the devices and strategies used to provide respiratory support of "sick" lungs. Multiple adjunctive agents have also been used in an attempt to mitigate the course of neonatal lung disease. There is considerable evidence supporting the use of one of the latter, exogenous surfactant therapy (discussed elsewhere in this issue). Many other therapies are currently being used as adjuncts to pulmonary management. The disorders we discuss include respiratory distress syndrome (RDS), chronic lung disease (CLD)/bronchopulmonary dysplasia (BPD), persistent pulmonary hypertension of the newborn (PPHN), meconium aspiration syndrome (MAS), and transient tachypnea of the newborn (TTN). We review the evidence that either supports or refutes the use of adjunctive therapies for these disorders. The gold standard to assess a given therapy is the randomized controlled trial (RCT). In this context, we discuss the support—or lack thereof—for multiple, commonly used therapies. Many of the therapies have been examined as systematic reviews by the Cochrane Neonatal Review Group. These reviews are noted in the references and can be easily accessed at the following

* Corresponding author.
E-mail address: thomas_wiswell@yahoo.com (T.E. Wiswell).

0095-5108/07/$ - see front matter © 2007 Elsevier Inc. All rights reserved.
doi:10.1016/j.clp.2006.12.006   *perinatology.theclinics.com*

website sponsored by the National Institute of Child Health and Human Development: www.nichd.nih.gov/cochrane/default.cfm.

Respiratory distress syndrome

Diuretic therapy

Lung edema and patent ductus arteriosus (PDA) may complicate RDS in preterm infants. These, along with renal insufficiency, are the major reasons that furosemide is the most common diuretic used in infants. Furosemide, which acts rapidly on the loop of Henle to inhibit active reabsorption of chloride, leads to active reabsorption of sodium. In addition, furosemide has a direct effect on reabsorption of lung fluid and can improve the lung function for a short period. The half-life of furosemide in term infants is about 8 hours, but it may be as long as 24 hours in preterm infants. Prolonged use increases renal loss of sodium and potassium and also urinary calcium excretion and the risk for renal calcium deposition. Early use of furosemide is associated with increased incidence of PDA in preterm infants because it stimulates the production of prostaglandin E2 from the kidneys. Repeated use of this therapy in preterm infants increases the risk for ototoxicity, and it can also enhance the risk for aminoglycoside ototoxicity [1]. Bumetanide is another loop diuretic with a mechanism of action similar to furosemide but is more potent and probably less ototoxic. It can also cause significant urinary losses of sodium, chloride, and calcium, however. The experience with bumetanide is limited in neonates [1]. Any type of diuretic therapy could promote excessive water loss and hypovolemia, potentially leading to hemodynamic instability. A systematic review of the use of diuretics for RDS in preterm infants has shown that such therapy has no effect on meaningful outcomes, including mortality, CLD, duration of mechanical ventilation and oxygen supplementation, and length of hospitalization [2]. All six trials included in this review were conducted before the era of antenatal steroid and surfactant replacement therapies. There is no current evidence to support the routine use of furosemide or any other diuretics in preterm infants who have RDS.

Opioid therapy

Ventilation is a potentially painful intervention. Neonates demonstrate increased sensitivity to pain, potentially affecting clinical and neurodevelopmental outcomes. Bellù and colleagues [3] performed a systematic review of opioid use in this population. They found no significant differences in important outcomes (mortality, duration of mechanical ventilation, and long- and short-term neurodevelopmental outcomes) and concluded there was insufficient evidence to recommend routine use of opioids in mechanically ventilated neonates.

Intravenous midazolam therapy

Sedation is commonly used in infants requiring respiratory support. The most common agent used is midazolam. Ng and colleagues [4] assessed the use of this agent in clinical trials. They found no particular advantages with this agent compared with placebo or morphine. In fact, there were increased adverse outcomes with midazolam use, including lower blood pressure, death, longer hospitalization, intracranial hemorrhages, and periventricular leukomalacia. We cannot recommend use of midazolam in ventilated preterm infants.

Neuromuscular paralytic therapy

Because ventilated newborn infants breathing asynchronously with mechanical ventilation are at risk for complications, neuromuscular relaxing agents have been used to abolish spontaneous breathing efforts. A review of such therapy has found it to potentially decrease the frequency of air leaks and intracranial bleeding [5]. Because of the uncertainty concerning long-term pulmonary and neurologic effects, however, routine use of these agents is not recommended.

Chronic lung disease

Chronic lung disease in premature infants is the "great constipator" of NICUs. Over the past two decades, success in lowering mortality among increasingly premature infants has resulted in a substantial proportion of these babies developing CLD and requiring prolonged pulmonary support. As has been done in most investigations, we define CLD as the need for supplemental oxygen at either 28 days of life or at 36 weeks' postmenstrual age (PMA), although there is considerable debate as to a consensus definition. Most of the adjunctive therapies used among preterm infants who have respiratory distress are given with the hope they will prevent or mitigate the course of CLD.

Diuretic therapy

The loop diuretic furosemide, the distal tubule diuretic thiazide, and the potassium-sparing diuretic spironolactone are all commonly used in preterm infants who have evolving or established CLD. These agents are administered parenterally, enterally, or by inhaled aerosol. These drugs are given to reduce alveolar and intersitial lung edema and to improve pulmonary mechanics. Despite their widespread use in this population, there are surprisingly few data assessing the value of these therapies. Additionally, their use frequently results in large urinary losses of electrolytes (sodium, potassium, and chloride) and minerals (calcium). As a consequence, alkalotic infants who have nephrocalcinosis and require supplemental electrolytes are frequently observed. Moreover, there is potential for hearing loss from these potent agents. Systematic reviews of diuretic therapy [6–8] indicate short-term improvement in pulmonary function. This finding does not translate to any substantial ability to decrease ventilator settings or to decrease the duration of mechanical ventilation. Overall, there are no long-term benefits of these therapies (no decrease in mortality, duration of ventilation, duration of oxygen use, or duration of hospitalization). Of all the adjunctive therapies used in ventilated newborns, diuretic therapy is the one most abused without evidence of substantive benefit.

Methylxanthine therapy

The methylxanthines (aminophylline, theophylline, and caffeine) have been used for more than three decades to treat apnea of prematurity [9]. This widespread use is based entirely on the reports of the short-term outcomes, and to date there are no data on the long term effects, including safety. In a systematic review of 192 infants from five trials, there was a reduction in recurrent apnea and the use of mechanical ventilation in the first 2 to 7 days of methylxanthine use [10]. The meta-analysis of six trials to study the prophylactic use of methylxanthine treatment for successful extubation [11] observed a 27% absolute reduction in the incidence of failed extubation. This benefit was observed only in babies less than 1000 g and those less than a week old. The advantages were lost if babies were less than 1000 g and more than a week of age, or 1000 to 1250 g who had previously failed extubation.

In addition, theophylline [12] and caffeine [13] have positive short-term effects on pulmonary mechanics in infants who have BPD, decreasing lung resistance and increasing compliance. These effects have only been studied for short periods of time (≤ 4 days), however, and there are no trials assessing whether there might be longer-term benefits of either agent.

Caffeine (usually in a form of caffeine citrate) is the preferred methylxanthine because of its wide therapeutic index with few side effects. Schmidt and colleagues [14] recently reported the short-term outcome "at neonatal discharge" of 2006 preterm infants who had birth weights between 500 and 1250 g. This multicenter, double-blind study, known as the CAP (Caffeine for Apnea of Prematurity) trial, demonstrated that caffeine reduced the durations of supplemental oxygen therapy, continuous positive airway pressure, and mechanical ventilation. Treated infants were less likely to have BPD, defined as need for supplemental oxygen at 36 weeks' PMA. Unexpectedly, caffeine therapy was also found to be associated with a reduction in the risk for PDA requiring pharmacologic or surgical closure. This large study also provides some reassurance that caffeine did not increase the incidence of neonatal complications, including necrotizing enterocolitis and ultrasonographic evidence of brain injury. One must recognize, however, that these published outcomes are not the primary outcome measure (which is to address the long-term safety of this commonly used therapy by follow-up at 18 months' corrected age). Clinicians should await the final report before drawing any conclusions.

Beta receptor agonist therapy

Bronchial hyperresponsiveness may be found in premature neonates who have RDS or those who have CLD. Assisted ventilation may aggravate this response. Bronchodilators, such as beta receptor agonists, are potentially attractive therapies for premature infants who have RDS or CLD. These agents may potentially widen small airways in infants who have compromised lungs. Denjean and colleagues [15] assessed the effect of albuterol (salbutamol) in preventing CLD. They found no evidence that albuterol reduces mortality or CLD at 28 days in preterm infants at risk for developing CLD (the study did not report outcomes for CLD at 36 weeks' PMA). Moreover, they did not demonstrate earlier weaning from respiratory support with albuterol or any decrease in the duration of oxygen supplementation. Additionally, albuterol (oral, intravenous, or inhalational) is commonly used in babies who have actual CLD. Nevertheless, to date there are no RCTs assessing important clinical outcomes following the use of bronchodilators in the treatment of CLD (eg, mortality, duration of oxygen use, CLD at 36 weeks, and so forth) [16]. Multiple short-term studies have assessed immediate changes in pulmonary mechanics (compliance, resistance) following the use of albuterol [16]. Several indicate that infants who have CLD may have improvement, no change, or even worsening of these parameters [17]. Whether beta receptor agonists are useful in treating CLD thus remains an unanswered question.

Anticholinergic therapy

Ipratropium bromide, a muscarinic antagonist, has some bronchodilatory activity and has been used to treat neonates who have CLD. The limited data available essentially consist of case reports following short-term use of the agent [18–21]. The results are mixed, with some demonstrating positive effects and some indicating either no or negative effects. Without supportive large RCTs, anticholinergic agents cannot be recommended in the management of CLD.

Cromolyn sodium therapy

Cromolyn sodium is a mast-cell stabilizer that also inhibits neutrophil activation and chemotaxis. As such, it could help regulate the inflammatory processes in the lung. Two small RCTs have been performed to assess whether early use of this substance can prevent CLD [22,23]. In neither study was there a difference in mortality or CLD (at 28 days or 36 weeks' PMA). Currently, there are no RCTs assessing the use of cromolyn sodium in the treatment of CLD. The limited data available consist of short-term case reports, which did not examine mortality or duration of ventilation, oxygen therapy, or hospitalization [24,25].

Vitamin A therapy

Vitamin A is involved in the regulation and promotion of growth and differentiation of multiple cells. Additionally, it maintains the integrity of the epithelial cells of the respiratory tract. Low serum concentrations of vitamin A in preterm infants have been associated with an increased risk for developing CLD. Several RCTs have assessed whether using supplemental vitamin A might prevent the development of CLD [26,27]. Supplementing very low birth weight infants with vitamin A is associated with a significant reduction in death or oxygen requirement at 1 month of age. Additionally, among infants of birth weights less than 1000 g, vitamin A supplementation is associated with a significantly decreased incidence of oxygen need among survivors at 36 weeks.

Vitamin E therapy

Vitamin E consists of several types of tocopherols, which have antioxidant activity. As a scavenger of free radicals, vitamin E could potentially limit processes that lead to CLD. The agent has been extensively studied in preterm infants with the hope that it could help prevent oxygen-related damage to multiple organs. A systematic review of the vitamin E trials in this population indicates that supplementation with this substance does not decrease the incidence of CLD [28].

Superoxide dismutase therapy

There has been hope that the antioxidant superoxide dismutase (SOD) could ameliorate oxygen free radical injury to the lungs of preterm infants. Two small RCTs have been performed assessing the effects of SOD in preventing CLD [29,30]. Unfortunately, in neither trial was there such a benefit. The use of SOD in premature infants thus cannot be recommended at this time.

Indomethacin and ibuprofen therapy

Presence of a PDA has been associated with a greater risk for CLD in premature infants [31]. Indomethacin is a cyclo-oxygenase inhibitor that has been a mainstay in treating or preventing PDAs over the past 25 years [32,33]. It is reasonable to think that a drug regimen that prevents PDA should, accordingly, reduce CLD in this population. The largest RCT to date assessing outcomes following prophylaxis with indomethacin, the international Trial of Indomethacin Prophylaxis in Preterms (TIPP) [33], found a significant decrease in the frequency of PDA following indomethacin therapy. There was no decrease in the incidence of CLD, however; in fact, there was not even a trend toward less CLD. This finding is true for virtually all RCTs that have assessed this therapy [32].

Side effects of indomethacin include potential organ damage from reduced blood flow to the brain, kidneys, or intestinal tract. Ibuprofen, another cyclo-oxygenase inhibitor, has been shown to be effective in PDA closure without reducing blood flow velocity to the brain, gut, or kidneys. The latter agent has also been assessed in RCTs with results similar to those seen with indomethacin; neither a significant reduction nor even a trend toward reduction of CLD was observed [34].

Corticosteroid therapy

Systemic and inhalational corticosteroids have long been used to prevent or treat CLD in preterm infants [35–39]. These therapies have been given early (<96 hours of age) [35] or moderately early (7–14 days of age) [36] with the hope of preventing CLD. Additionally, corticosteroids have been given delayed or late (>3 weeks of age) [37] for treatment of the disorder. Both early and moderately early systemic corticosteroids significantly reduce the incidence of CLD at either 28 days of age or 36 weeks' PMA. Following moderately early treatment, there was a reduction in death through 28 days of age but not thereafter. No reductions in mortality were seen following early treatment. Unfortunately, these apparent benefits come at a price: more adverse outcomes, including hypertension, hyperglycemia, gastrointestinal bleeding, hypertrophic cardiomyopathy, and infection [35,36]. Moreover, in the trials that have reported late outcomes following early treatment with systemic corticosteroids, several adverse neurologic effects were significantly more likely to be found at follow-up examinations of survivors who had received the agents, including developmental delay, cerebral palsy, and abnormal neurologic examinations [35]. The limited data from studies giving these drugs moderately early did not show evidence of an increase in adverse neurologic outcomes [36]. Delayed or late use of these agents for treatment of CLD had no effect on mortality and had a borderline effect on decreasing CLD at 36 weeks' PMA [37]. Treatment at greater than 3 weeks of age did not significantly increase the occurrence of infection, hyperglycemia, or gastrointestinal complications, although hypertension was significantly more common among those receiving the agents. Moreover, although there was an increased rate of abnormal neurologic examination among those receiving delayed therapy, the rates of cerebral palsy and major neurosensory disabilities were not increased.

A systematic review of inhalational versus systemic corticosteroids to prevent CLD has revealed a borderline increase in the incidence of CLD at 36 weeks' PMA [38]. Moreover, inhalational corticosteroids are no more effective than systemically administered drugs when used to treat CLD (36 weeks' PMA) [39]. There are no long-term neurodevelopmental outcomes available from the studies of inhalational corticosteroids when used either prophylactically or therapeutically for CLD.

In view of concerns about long- and short-term adverse effects, the Committee on Fetus and Newborn of the American Academy of Pediatrics has recommended that corticosteroids not be routinely used to prevent or treat CLD [40].

Erythromycin therapy

Ureaplasma urealyticum is a common type of infection that has been implicated in the pathogenesis of CLD, although this has not been proven [41]. Nevertheless, two small RCTs have been performed to assess the efficacy of the antibiotic erythromycin in the prevention of CLD in intubated preterm infants at risk for, or colonized or infected with, this organism [42,43]. In these trials, there was no effect on death or on the development of CLD.

Fluid restriction

Several studies have found an association between relative fluid restriction and the prevention of CLD [44]. The belief is that standard fluid therapy may lead to the development of PDA or to excessive lung fluid, both contributing to the development of CLD. This is a particularly difficult area to assess in preterm infants, because there are major differences across the spectrum of preterm infants in their body fluid composition and fluid losses. The opinion of what represents fluid restriction in very low birth weight infants varies widely. Anecdotal data continue to accumulate, seemingly supporting the potential benefits of relative fluid restriction among preterm infants [45]. A systematic review of fluid restriction has not found this management to decrease CLD, however [44]. Further RCTs of sufficient size are needed to determine whether the incidence of CLD can be reduced by controlling fluid and electrolyte administration.

Inhaled nitric oxide therapy

Inhaled nitric oxide (iNO) is effective in term infants who have hypoxemic respiratory failure (see later discussion). iNO is a potent pulmonary vasodilator. Some premature infants who have RDS have increased pulmonary vascular resistance and elevated pulmonary artery pressure, factors that likely impede oxygenation. A recent systematic review assessed the RCTs that have investigated whether iNO may be of benefit in the preterm population [46]. The latter review, however, did not include two recently published RCTs [47,48]. The systematic review found no improvement in major outcomes (mortality before 36 weeks' PMA or CLD at 36 weeks' PMA). One of these trials indicated that iNO initiated in non-Caucasian infants of birth weight 500 to 799 g would increase survival without CLD at 36 weeks' PMA [47]. In the other trial, iNO was initiated at a mean of 31 hours of age [48]. Overall, in the latter trial there was no difference in mortality or CLD at 36 weeks' PMA. There seemed to be some benefit, however, among infants who had birth weights between 1000 and 1250 g. In light of the expense of iNO, the lack of long-term follow-up data, and no consistent positive results, the authors believe that routine use of the therapy in preterm infants is not justifiable at this time and should be limited to clinical trials.

Oxygen therapy

Supplemental oxygen is the most commonly used adjunctive therapy to mechanical ventilatory support in newborn infants who have pulmonary problems. The ultimate goal of oxygen therapy is to achieve adequate tissue oxygenation without creating oxygen toxicity and oxidative stress. In addition to the inspired oxygen, tissue oxygenation depends on several other factors, including gas exchange mechanisms within the lungs, oxygen carrying capacity of the blood, cardiac output, and local tissue edema or ischemia. Optimizing the latter factors may allow adequate oxygenation with the use of minimal supplemental oxygen. Direct exposure to high concentrations of oxygen can damage the pulmonary epithelium. This has been recognized as an important factor in the pathogenesis of CLD since its first description by Northway and colleagues [49]. Even if the inspired oxygen fraction is not high, oxidative stress (defined as an imbalance between pro- and antioxidant forces) can occur, especially in the preterm infants who are more vulnerable to the harmful effects of free oxygen radicals [50]. To date there are insufficient data to suggest the optimal oxygen level for preterm infants receiving oxygen therapy. There are no completed RCTs that have adequately addressed this issue. Published observational studies suggest that in comparison with the liberal approach of attempting to keep high oxygen saturation values (measured by pulse oximetry), the restrictive approach of accepting lower oxygen saturation values is associated with decreased incidences of retinopathy of prematurity (ROP) and CLD, without a concomitant increased risk for mortality [51,52]. The follow-up information available from one of these studies showed that the restrictive approach of oxygen therapy did not increase the risk for cerebral palsy [51], and more relevantly, it was not associated with any disadvantages in intellectual skills, academic achievements, adaptive functioning, or behavior [53]. In contrast, a retrospective analysis of observational data involving 891 babies of less than 30 weeks' gestation admitted to two neonatal units that used different pulse oximetry limits (80%–92% versus 92%–97%) revealed the incidence of severe ROP (stage 3 or greater) to be significantly higher in the unit that used lower oxygen saturation limits (13% versus 6%), although no difference was seen in the incidence of ROP that required surgery [54]. The lack of knowledge and ongoing uncertainty as to what is the optimal oxygenation for newborn infants has led to wide variation of policies on oxygen monitoring and therapy in neonatal nurseries [55,56]. As Silverman [57] noted, observational studies over the past 50 years have gotten us nowhere. The only way to resolve the uncertainties and controversies of oxygen monitoring and therapy is to conduct well-designed RCTs [57].

In response to the growing demand to resolve the uncertainty surrounding oxygen therapy in very preterm babies, an international collaborative effort has been mounted since 2003 to conduct large, multicenter, masked RCTs to address the issue of the most appropriate oxygen saturation target for very premature infants. Infants less than 28 weeks' gestation are eligible for these trials if they are less than 24 hours of age. It is estimated that more than 5000 babies will be enrolled and randomized into one of two groups, in which the concentration of inspired oxygen is varied to maintain either a low oxygen saturation range (85%–89%) versus a high range (91%–95%). The subjects will be kept in these groups until they are breathing room air or until 36 weeks' PMA. The research outcomes will include: (1) death or severe neurosensory disability at a corrected age of 2 years, (2) the need for invasive intervention for ROP, (3) the need for supplemental oxygen or respiratory support at 36 weeks' PMA, (4) the incidence of PDA and NEC, and (5) growth parameters (eg, weight, length, and head circumference) at 36 weeks' PMA and 2 years of age. The raw individual patient data from all the trials will be combined to detect small differences in outcomes.

Until the uncertainties and controversies about oxygen therapy and its monitoring are resolved, clinicians should follow the words of wisdom by Comroe and colleagues [58] in 1945: "The clinician must bear in mind that oxygen is a drug and must be used in accordance with well recognized pharmacologic principles; ie, because it has certain toxic effects and is not completely harmless (as widely believed in clinical circles) it should be given only in the lowest dosage or concentration required by the particular patient."

Persistent pulmonary hypertension of the newborn

Inhaled nitric oxide therapy

PPHN is a frustrating disorder for clinicians and parents. This life-threatening illness had a mortality rate of greater than 75% as recently as the late 1970s. Over the past decade, some of the most comprehensive RCTs ever performed in neonatology have addressed the use of iNO in managing PPHN [46]. These have assessed whether treatment of hypoxemic term and near-term newborn infants with iNO improves oxygenation and reduces the rates of death or the requirement for extracorporeal membrane oxygenation (ECMO), or affects long term neurodevelopmental outcomes. The systematic review of the iNO trials [46] has reached the following conclusions: (1) iNO does not decrease mortality, and (2) iNO significantly decreases the need for ECMO. Follow-up studies to date have not found any increases in neurodevelopmental outcomes in infants treated with iNO versus controls.

Meconium aspiration syndrome

Corticosteroid therapy

Meconium aspiration syndrome (MAS) may cause severe respiratory distress, occurring generally in term or postterm neonates. There may be relatively high morbidity and mortality. A profound inflammatory response to meconium and its constituents is noted within hours of aspiration [59]. Because of their anti-inflammatory properties, corticosteroids could potentially be of benefit in the management of MAS. To date, two RCTs have assessed the role of this therapy [60,61]. The results of these trials demonstrate no differences in the following outcomes: mortality, oxygen dependency at 28 days, duration of mechanical ventilation, pulmonary air leaks, or duration of hospitalization. The duration of oxygen therapy was significantly longer among infants receiving corticosteroids. Nevertheless, because a total of only 85 patients were enrolled in these two trials, there is likely insufficient power to determine whether there is a role for this therapy. A large RCT, including assessment of acute and long-term adverse effects, would be required to adequately assess efficacy [62].

Transient tachypnea of the newborn

Diuretic therapy

Transient tachypnea of the newborn ("wet lung") results from delayed clearance of fetal lung fluid. It is a common reason for admission of term or near-term infants to NICUs. The condition is particularly common following delivery by cesarean section. Conventional treatment consists of supplemental oxygen as needed. Many affected infants are assessed for possible infection and placed on antibiotics. Hospitalization may be prolonged because of persistent tachypnea and delays in establishing enteral feeding. Occasionally, some infants who have TTN require continuous positive airway pressure, mechanical ventilation, and even ECMO. Hastening the clearance of lung liquid could potentially shorten the duration of the clinical manifestations and reduce complications. To date, there is only one RCT that has assessed the use of a diuretic (furosemide) in the management of TTN [63]. Compared with infants in the control group, the furosemide-treated group demonstrated no significant differences in the duration of tachypnea or in the length of hospitalization. Of note, however, is that in the trial furosemide was administered orally. Further trials assessing furosemide or other diuretics given either intravenously or inhalationally might result in different outcomes.

Summary

Respiratory disorders continue to be major problems among sick neonates. The disorders carry the potential for mortality and major morbidity. Not all infants do well with conventional pulmonary support, and most clinicians often use other therapeutic modalities. As with much of neonatal care, many therapeutic agents have made their way into our armamentarium unimpeded by adequate assessment for safety or efficacy. When one carefully examines the evidence for the many adjunctive therapies used for newborn lung diseases, there is little to no basis to support the use of the vast majority of them. We owe it to our patients and their families to practice evidence-based medicine.

References

[1] Hey E, editor. Neonatal formulary. 4th edition. London: BMJ Books; 2003.
[2] Brion LP, Soll RF. Diuretics for respiratory distress syndrome in preterm infants. Cochrane Database Syst Rev 2001;2:CD001454.
[3] Bellù R, de Waal KA, Zanini R. Opioids for neonates receiving mechanical ventilation. Cochrane Database Syst Rev 2005;1:CD004212.
[4] Ng E, Taddio A, Ohlsson A. Intravenous midazolam infusion for sedation of infants in the neonatal intensive care unit. Cochrane Database Syst Rev 2003;1:CD002052.
[5] Cools F, Offringa M. Neuromuscular paralysis for newborn infants receiving mechanical ventilation. Cochrane Database Syst Rev 2005;2:CD002773.
[6] Brion LP, Primhak RA, Ambrosio-Perez I. Diuretics acting on the distal renal tubule for preterm infants with (or developing) chronic lung disease. Cochrane Database Syst Rev 2002;1: CD001817.
[7] Brion LP, Primhak RA. Intravenous or enteral loop diuretics for preterm infants with (or developing) chronic lung disease. Cochrane Database Syst Rev 2002;1:CD001453.
[8] Brion LP, Primhak RA, Yong W. Aerosolized diuretics for preterm infants with (or developing) chronic lung disease. Cochrane Database Syst Rev 2006;3:CD001694.
[9] Weinberg BA, Bealer BK. The world of caffeine: the science and culture of the world's most popular drug. New York: Routledge; 2002.
[10] Henderson-Smart DJ, Steer P. Methylxanthine treatment for apnea in preterm infants. Cochrane Database Syst Rev 2001;3:CD000140.
[11] Henderson-Smart DJ, Davis PG. Prophylactic methylxanthines for extubation in preterm infants. Cochrane Database Syst Rev 2003;1:CD000139.
[12] Kao LC, Durand DJ, Phillips BL, et al. Oral theophylline and diuretics improve pulmonary mechanics in infants with bronchopulmonary dysplasia. J Pediatr 1987;111:439–44.
[13] Davis JM, Bhutani VK, Stefano JL, et al. Changes in pulmonary mechanics following caffeine administration in infants with bronchopulmonary dysplasia. Pediatr Pulmonol 1989; 6:49–52.
[14] Schmidt B, Roberts RS, Davis P, et al. Caffeine therapy for apnea of prematurity. N Engl J Med 2006;354:2112–21.
[15] Denjean A, Paris-Llado J, Zupan V, et al. Inhaled salbutamol and beclomethasone for preventing broncho-pulmonary dysplasia: a randomised double-blind study. Eur J Pediatr 1998;157:926–31.
[16] Ng GY, da Silva O, Ohlsson A. Bronchodilators for the prevention and treatment of chronic lung disease in preterm infants. Cochrane Database Syst Rev 2001;3:CD003214.
[17] Holt WJ, Greenspan JS, Wiswell TE, et al. Pulmonary response to an inhaled bronchodilator in chronically ventilated preterm Infants with suspected airway reactivity. Respir Care 1995; 40:145–51.
[18] Wilkie RA, Bryan MH. Effect of bronchodilators on airway resistance in ventilator-dependent neonates with chronic lung disease. J Pediatr 1987;111:278–82.
[19] Brundage KL, Mohsini KG, Froese AB, et al. Bronchodilator response to ipratropium bromide in infants with bronchopulmonary dysplasia. Am Rev Respir Dis 1990;142:1137–42.
[20] Yuksel B, Greenough A, Green S. Paradoxical response to nebulized ipratropium bromide in pre-term infants asymptomatic at follow-up. Respir Med 1991;85:189–94.

[21] Yuksel B, Greenough A. Ipratropium bromide for symptomatic preterm infants. Eur J Pediatr 1991;150:854–7.

[22] Watterberg KL, Murphy S. Failure of cromolyn sodium to reduce the incidence of broncho-pulmonary dysplasia: a pilot study. Pediatrics 1993;91:803–6.

[23] Viscardi RM, Hasday JD, Gumpper KF, et al. Cromolyn sodium prophylaxis inhibits pulmonary proinflammatory cytokines in infants at high risk for bronchopulmonary dysplasia. Am J Respir Crit Care Med 1997;156:1523–9.

[24] Yamamoto C, Kojima T, Sasai M, et al. Disodium cromoglycate in the treatment of bronchopulmonary dysplasia. Acta Paediatr Jpn 1992;34:589–91.

[25] Kassur-Siemienska B, Milewska-Bobula B, Dmenska H, et al. Longitudinal study of children with bronchopulmonary dysplasia treated with disodium cromoglycate. Med Wieku Rozwoj 2003;7(3 Suppl 1):343–50.

[26] Tyson JE, Wright LL, Oh W, et al. Vitamin A supplementation for extremely-low-birth-weight infants. N Engl J Med 1999;340:1962–8.

[27] Darlow BA, Graham PJ. Vitamin A supplementation for preventing morbidity and mortality in very low birthweight infants. Cochrane Database Syst Rev 2002;4:CD000501.

[28] Brion LP, Bell EF, Rughuveer TS. Vitamin E supplementation for prevention of morbidity and mortality in preterm infants. Cochrane Database Syst Rev 2003;4:CD003665.

[29] Rosenfeld W, Evans H, Concepcion L, et al. Prevention of bronchopulmonary dysplasia by administration of bovine superoxide dismutase in preterm infants with respiratory distress syndrome. J Pediatr 1984;105:781–5.

[30] Davis JM, Rosenfeld WN, Richter SE, et al. Safety and pharmacokinetics of multiple doses of recombinant human CuZn superoxide dismutase administered intratracheally to premature neonates with respiratory distress syndrome. Pediatrics 1997;100:24–30.

[31] Bancalari E. Changes in the pathogenesis and prevention of chronic lung disease of prematurity. Am J Perinatol 2001;18:1–9.

[32] Fowlie PW, Davis PG. Prophylactic intravenous indomethacin for preventing mortality and morbidity in preterm infants. Cochrane Database Syst Rev 2002;3:CD000174.

[33] Schmidt B, Davis P, Moddemann D, et al. Long-term effects of indomethacin prophylaxis in extremely-low-birth-weight infants. N Engl J Med 2001;344:1966–72.

[34] Shah SS, Ohlsson A. Ibuprofen for the prevention of patent ductus arteriosus in preterm and/or low birth weight infants. Cochrane Database Syst Rev 2006;1:CD004213.

[35] Halliday HL, Ehrenkranz RA, Doyle LW. Early postnatal (<96 hours) corticosteroids for preventing chronic lung disease in preterm infants. Cochrane Database Syst Rev 2003;1:CD001146.

[36] Halliday HL, Ehrenkranz RA, Doyle LW. Moderately early (7–14 days) postnatal cortico-steroids for preventing chronic lung disease in preterm infants. Cochrane Database Syst Rev 2003;1:CD001144.

[37] Halliday HL, Ehrenkranz RA, Doyle LW. Delayed (>3 weeks) postnatal corticosteroids for chronic lung disease in preterm infants. Cochrane Database Syst Rev 2003;1:CD001145.

[38] Shah SS, Ohlsson A, Halliday H, et al. Inhaled versus systemic corticosteroids for preventing chronic lung disease in ventilated very low birth weight preterm neonates. Cochrane Database Syst Rev 2003;1:CD002058.

[39] Shah SS, Ohlsson A, Halliday H, et al. Inhaled versus systemic corticosteroids for the treatment of chronic lung disease in ventilated very low birth weight preterm infants. Cochrane Database Syst Rev 2003;2:CD002057.

[40] Committee on Fetus and Newborn. Postnatal corticosteroids to prevent or treat chronic lung disease in preterm infants. Pediatrics 2002;109:330–8.

[41] Mabanta CG, Pryhuber GS, Weinberg GA, et al. Erythromycin for the prevention of chronic lung disease in intubated preterm infants at risk for, or colonized or infected with Urea-plasma urealyticum. Cochrane Database Syst Rev 2003;4:CD003744.

[42] Jonsson B, Rylander M, Faxelius G. Ureaplasma urealyticum, erythromycin and respiratory morbidity in high-risk preterm neonates. Acta Paediatr 1998;87:1079–84.

[43] Lyon AJ, McColm J, Middlemist L, et al. Randomised trial of erythromycin on the development of chronic lung disease in preterm infants. Arch Dis Child Fetal Neonatal Ed 1998;78: F10–4.

[44] Bell EF, Acarregui MJ. Restricted versus liberal water intake for preventing morbidity and mortality in preterm infants. Cochrane Database Syst Rev 2001;3:CD000503.

[45] Oh W, Poindexter BB, Perritt R, et al. Association between fluid intake and weight loss during the first ten days of life and risk of bronchopulmonary dysplasia in extremely low birth weight infants. J Pediatr 2005;147:786–90.

[46] Barrington KJ, Finer NN. Nitric oxide for respiratory failure in infants born at or near term. Cochrane Database Syst Rev 2006;4:CD000399.

[47] Ballard RA, Truog WE, Cnaan A, et al. Inhaled nitric oxide in preterm infants undergoing mechanical ventilation. N Engl J Med 2006;355:343–53.

[48] Kinsella JP, Cutter GR, Walsh WF, et al. Early inhaled nitric oxide therapy in premature infants with respiratory failure. N Engl J Med 2006;355:354–64.

[49] Northway WH Jr, Rosan RC, Porter DY. Pulmonary disease following respirator therapy of hyaline membrane disease. Bronchopulmonary dysplasia. N Engl J Med 1967;276:357–68.

[50] Saugstad OD. Brochopulmonary dysplasia-oxidative stress and oxidants. Semin Neonatol 2003;8:39–49.

[51] Tin W, Milligan DWA, Pennefather P, et al. Pulse oximetry, severe retinopathy, and outcome at one year in babies of less than 28 weeks gestation. Arch Dis Child 2001;84:F106–10.

[52] Sun SC. Relation of target SpO2 levels and clinical outcome in ELBW infants on supplemental oxygen. Pediatr Res 2002;51:A350.

[53] Bradley S, Anderson K, Tin W, et al. Early oxygen exposure and outcome at 10 years in babies of less than 28 weeks. Pediatr Res 2004;55:A373.

[54] Poets C, Arand J, Hummler H, et al. Retinopathy of prematurity: a comparison between two centers aiming for different pulse oximetry saturation levels. Biol Neonate 2003;4:A267.

[55] Vijayakumar E, Ward GJ, Bullock CE, et al. Pulse oximetry in infants < 1500 gm at birth on supplemental oxygen: a national survey. J Perinatol 1997;17:341–5.

[56] Tin W, Wariyar U. Giving small babies oxygen: 50 years of uncertainty. Semin Neonatol 2002;7:361–7.

[57] Silverman WA. A cautionary tale about supplemental oxygen: the albatross of neonatal medicine. Pediatrics 2004;113:394–6.

[58] Comroe JH Jr, Dripps RD, Dumke PR, et al. Oxygen toxicity: the effect of inhalation of high concentrations of oxygen for twenty-four hours on normal men at sea level and at a simulated altitude of 18,000 feet. JAMA 1945;128:710–7.

[59] Cleary GM, Wiswell TE. Meconium-stained amniotic fluid and the meconium aspiration syndrome. An update. Pediatr Clin North Am 1998;45:511–29.

[60] Yeh TF, Srinivasan G, Harris V, et al. Hydrocortisone therapy in meconium aspiration syndrome: a controlled study. J Pediatr 1977;90:140–3.

[61] Wu JM, Yeh TF, Wang JY, et al. The role of pulmonary inflammation in the development of pulmonary hypertension in newborn with meconium aspiration syndrome. Pediatr Pulmonol Suppl 1999;18:205–8.

[62] Ward M, Sinn J. Steroid therapy for meconium aspiration syndrome in newborn infants. Cochrane Database Syst Rev 2003;4:CD003485.

[63] Wiswell TE, Rawlings JS, Smith FR, et al. Effect of furosemide on the clinical course of transient tachypnea of the newborn. Pediatrics 1985;75:908–10.

ELSEVIER
SAUNDERS

CLINICS IN
PERINATOLOGY

Clin Perinatol 34 (2007) 205–217

Long-Term Outcomes: What Should the Focus Be?

Judy L. Aschner, MD[a,b,*], Michele C. Walsh, MD[c,d]

[a]Department of Pediatrics and The Vanderbilt Kennedy Center, Vanderbilt University Medical Center, Nashville, TN 37232-9544, USA
[b]Division of Neonatology, Vanderbilt Children's Hospital, 11111 Doctor's Office Tower, 2200 Children's Way, Nashville, TN 37232-9544, USA
[c]Case Western Reserve University, Cleveland, OH 44106-6010, USA
[d]NICU, Rainbow Babies and Childrens Hospital, Division of Neonatology, Mailstop 6010, 11100 Euclid Avenue, Cleveland, OH 44106-6010, USA

Of all therapies used in the neonatal period, none has been as extensively studied as surfactant replacement therapy (SRT) for the prevention and treatment of respiratory distress syndrome (RDS) of the premature [1]. More than 400 clinical trials have evaluated the optimal timing, the optimal dosing, and the overall efficacy of different surfactant preparations. Many of the largest clinical trials were performed in the late 1980s and early 1990s. These early trials focused primarily on short-term outcomes, such as RDS mortality and the incidence of air leak. Despite this limitation, there is little debate about the merits of these early clinical trials or the efficacy of SRT. In many respects, the surfactant trials of the 1980s and early 1990s represent the finest efforts of the neonatal scientific community and are excellent examples of high-impact translational research that have resulted in a fundamental change in clinical practice. In the intervening decade and a half, however, there have been significant changes in the demographics of the patients for whom we care, as well as the antenatal and postnatal management of preterm infants. The neonatology community has also matured in its thinking and expectations about relevant biologic and clinical endpoints in randomized controlled trials. Thus, it is timely to address the question

This work was supported by Grants HL07551, HL06857 and ES013730-01 from the National Institutes of Health and a grant from the Gerber Foundation.

* Corresponding author. Vanderbilt Children's Hospital, 11111 Doctor's Office Tower, 2200 Children's Way, Nashville, TN 37232-9544.

E-mail address: judy.aschner@vanderbilt.edu (J.L. Aschner).

of which short- and long-term outcomes future clinical trials of SRT or other neonatal respiratory interventions should be powered to detect.

Looking through the "retrospectoscope"

A review of the recent literature reveals an impressive number of randomized clinical trials, systematic reviews, and meta-analyses in neonatal medicine. Unfortunately, closer perusal exposes that most have focused only on short-term neonatal intensive care unit (NICU) outcomes. This is particularly true of clinical trials of respiratory management. The Cochrane library hosts at least eight systematic reviews of SRT, covering a breadth of clinical questions, including multiple versus single dose surfactant [2], prophylactic versus selective surfactant administration [3], early versus delayed selective surfactant treatment [4], and natural surfactant extract versus synthetic surfactant for neonatal RDS [5]. The early trials of SRT focused primarily upon short-term pulmonary responses and rarely examined outcomes beyond initial hospital discharge. A review by Morley and Davis [6] examined the major outcomes in 35 randomized placebo-controlled trials of SRT. Compared to the placebo group, infants who received SRT had fewer pneumothoraces, less pulmonary interstitial emphysema, lower 28-day mortality, and lower in-hospital mortality rates. Acute benefits attributed to SRT included improvements in oxygenation, reduction in mean airway pressure, but no effect on important intermediate-term outcomes such as bronchopulmonary dysplasia (BPD), intraventricular hemorrhage, retinopathy of prematurity, or length of hospital stay. As noted by Suresh and Soll [1], long-term outcomes have not been studied as comprehensively as short-term morbidity and mortality.

To assess the relative benefit versus harm of a therapy, however, it is essential to study its long-term efficacy and safety. In 2002, Sinn and colleagues [7] reviewed the neurodevelopmental outcomes at 1 and 2 years of age of infants enrolled in randomized controlled trials of SRT that reported these outcomes. In this systematic review, the main outcome measures were severe and mild disability at 1 and 2 years, plus the composite adverse outcome of death and/or severe disability. Among 13 RCT reporting neurodevelopmental outcomes, follow-up at 1 year of age was reported for 2218 treated and 2090 control infants; follow-up between 18 months and 2 years of age was reported for only 303 treated and 292 control infants. SRT was associated with a lower rate of mild disability at 1 year (OR 0.79; 95% CI 0.66–0.95), reduction in combined adverse outcome (death or severe disability) at 1 year (OR 0.8; 95% CI 0.72–0.89), but, perhaps secondary to lack of power, no differences were noted at 2 years.

There are obvious limitations to this meta-analysis that were pointed out by the authors themselves [7]. Lack of detailed data prevented analysis of disability rates based on birth weight or gestational age. Follow-up was limited to 2 years, by which time the sample size had decreased to 13% of the original data set. More subtle disabilities, such as learning difficulties, poor school performance, attention deficit disorders, behavioral problems, minor motor problems, and mild cerebral palsy may not be evident until school age and were not specifically evaluated. The authors were skeptical that new large randomized controlled trials of SRT would be carried out in the future.

That last prediction proved incorrect as a new synthetic surfactant, lucinactant, entered clinical trials. The initial publications describing two multinational randomized controlled trials reported only short-term outcomes [8,9]. The primary outcome measures included the rates of RDS at 24 hours and the rates of death related to RDS during the first 14 days after birth [8], and the incidence of being alive without BPD through 28 days of age [9]. Prespecified secondary outcomes included all-cause mortality rates at 28 days and 36 weeks, BPD rates, neuroimaging abnormalities, and rates of other complications of prematurity. One-year follow up assessments were built into the design for both trials, the results of which are currently in press.

Inadequate longer-term outcome data are not the only limitations when attempting to interpret the previously published SRT trials. Significant changes in neonatal care practices have occurred since the late 1980s and early 1990s when most RCTs of SRT were conducted. The evolution of care in this intervening time period included the resuscitation of younger and smaller preterm infants, changes in the style and sophistication of mechanical ventilation, and more frequent use of early continuous positive airway pressure. Perinatal care practices have also changed markedly since the 1980s with a higher rate of cesarean section and more routine use of antenatal steroids in pregnant women at high risk of preterm delivery. For example, in the intervening two decades, administration of antenatal steroids has increased from approximately 30% to over 70%. This single change in obstetric practice could have a profound effect on the response to SRT and alter the risk/benefit ratio for infants currently receiving SRT compared to those enrolled in the early randomized controlled trials. Thus, it is important to ponder the applicability and generalizability of the reported outcomes to the patients we currently treat with SRT.

This issue was raised by Morley and Davis [6], who noted that most trials excluded babies who had other complications of preterm birth, and many restricted enrollment to infants in a specific birth weight category or had a particular severity of lung disease. They illustrated their point with the original US Survanta trial [10] and the more recent European Curosurf trial [11]. The Survanta trial restricted enrollment to infants who had RDS with birth weights between 750 and 1750 g who required FiO_2 greater than 0.4 and were between 3 to 6 hours of age. Excluded were infants with hypotension, hypoglycemia, hyperglycemia, or seizures [10]. The Curosurf trial only enrolled infants with birth weights between 700 and 2000 g who received surfactant between 2 and 15 hours of life and had FiO_2 greater than 0.6 [11]. This represents approximately 10% of babies who have RDS [6]. Current clinical use of SRT is not nearly as selective.

Spotlight on the present

This brings us to the primary goal of this review: consideration of what population of infants we should be studying currently, and what outcomes should be targeted in future studies of SRT or other therapies focused on the respiratory outcomes of preterm infants. We must avoid the temptation to target enticing but unimportant end points, such as fall in FiO_2 or oxygenation index in the hours or days after an experimental intervention. Relevant primary outcomes might include BPD incidence and severity, the combined outcome of death or BPD, length of hospital stay, health services resource utilization and cost effectiveness, long-term neurodevelopmental outcome, long-term pulmonary outcome, and assessments of quality of life. The choice of primary outcome will obviously influence trial size and trial design. Numerous changes in clinical practices that have occurred in the postsurfactant era should also influence the study design of future surfactant trials as well as lend guidance to appropriate primary outcomes. These changes include less-frequent administration of surfactant as a prophylactic strategy in the delivery room, particularly for infants greater than 1000 g [12], and more aggressive use of noninvasive support, such as early nasal continuous positive airway pressure [13,14], although admittedly these changes in clinical practice have not themselves been subjected to the type of rigorous evaluation of safety and efficacy that must be advocated in future clinical trials.

It is time for careful consideration of the validity, relevance, and limitations of commonly targeted short- and long-term outcomes in neonatal clinical trials. The ideal primary outcomes are those that are objective, rather than subjective, occur with sufficient frequency to offer practical enrollment targets, and are important to the child's long-term quality of life. RDS mortality, for example, no longer serves as a relevant primary outcome. Death from RDS in the first or second week is an infrequent occurrence in contemporary NICUs. Death before discharge, although clearly objective and relevant, is influenced by comorbidities and ethical considerations and would be an applicable endpoint only for infants with birth weights of less than 800 g, because death occurs infrequently in larger preterm infants and is more often attributable to nonrespiratory causes.

Composite outcomes are frequently used in contemporary neonatal clinical trials. The value of such combined outcomes as death or BPD (or its counterpart, survival without BPD) becomes clear when considering an intervention that may increase the percentage of survivors that do not have BPD by increasing the mortality among the sickest or most vulnerable infants. Such composite outcomes also adjust for differences among centers in their willingness to withdraw support from infants who have a poor neurodevelopmental prognosis.

Although BPD cannot be considered a long-term outcome, the incidence of BPD remains a relevant endpoint for clinical trials of respiratory management in preterm infants. BPD is an important cause of morbidity and mortality and has been associated with prolonged and recurrent hospitalizations and linked to higher rates of other serious complications of prematurity [15]. Its incidence is high with 7000 to 10,000 new cases each year in the United States alone, and it has not been reduced by numerous interventions, including SRT. The prevalence of BPD has actually increased in the past decade as more extremely low birth weight infants survive to discharge. Long-term follow-up suggests that compared to gestational age-matched infants who do not have BPD, infants that have BPD have life-long alterations in lung function [16,17] and an increased incidence of cerebral palsy and neurodevelopmental delays [18,19]. However, the caveats to designing and powering a study based on a reduction in the incidence of BPD deserve discussion.

The incidence of BPD is highly birth weight– and gestational age–specific, occurring in less than 30% of infants with birth weights greater than 1000 g but in as many as 85% of those with birth weights less than 700 g [19]. Thus, studies targeting BPD rate as a primary outcome must, by design, enroll extremely low birth-weight infants. The diagnosis of BPD is highly subjective and influenced by local clinical practices, such as oxygen saturation targets [20]. Attempts to reduce the subjectivity of the diagnosis of BPD have gained momentum in recent years. Walsh and colleagues [21] examined the safety, reliability, and validity of implementing a physiologic definition of BPD [20] and the impact of this approach on the BPD rates among different NICUs. Noting that the outcome of BPD is confounded by center-specific criteria for supplemental oxygen administration, an effort was made to standardize the definition of BPD by administering an oxygen saturation monitoring test at 36 weeks postmenstrual age. Neonates receiving mechanical ventilation or FiO_2 greater than 0.3 were defined as having BPD without further testing. Those receiving FiO_2 of less than or equal to 0.3 underwent a stepwise reduction in supplemental oxygen to 21%. Those who maintained oxygen saturations of at least 88% for 60 minutes were considered to be without BPD, whereas those whose saturations fell to less than 88% met the physiologic definition of BPD. Approximately 7% of infants clinically treated with oxygen successfully passed the saturation-monitoring test in room air. The authors concluded that a physiologic definition of BPD is safe, feasible, reliable, and valid and improves the precision of the diagnosis of BPD. They further suggested that use of this standardized approach may be of benefit in future multicenter clinical trials [20].

A subsequent study conducted by the National Institute of Child Health and Human Development (NICHD) Neonatal Network prospectively tested the hypothesis that a physiologic definition of BPD would reduce variation in observed rates of BPD among centers [21]. This study enrolled 1598 infants with birth weights between 501 and 1250 g who remained hospitalized at 36 weeks postmenstrual age. Each infant was assigned an outcome with both a clinical definition and a physiologic definition of BPD. The clinical definition of BPD was oxygen supplementation at exactly 36 weeks postmenstrual age. Neonates requiring mechanical ventilation or FiO_2 greater than 0.3 with oxygen saturations between 90% and 96% were determined to have BPD and not tested further. Those receiving FiO_2 less than or equal to 0.3 with saturations greater than 96% underwent a room air challenge. A physiologic diagnosis of BPD was made if room air saturations fell to less than 90%; those who maintained saturations at least 90% in room air for 30 minutes were classified as not having BPD. Use of the physiologic definition reduced the overall BPD rate at 36 weeks from 35% to 25%. The impact of using a physiologic definition of BPD differed among centers; the reduction in BPD incidence ranged from 0% to 44%. Sixteen centers had a decrease in BPD rate, with only one center experiencing no change in its rate of BPD. This prospective study suggests that the use of a physiologic definition of BPD will reduce the overall rate of BPD and will likewise reduce the variation among centers [21].

The magnitude of the change in BPD rate when the physiologic definition is applied is comparable to the magnitude of treatment effects seen in some clinical trials. This fact alone suggests that use of a physiologic definition of BPD will facilitate the measurement of BPD as an outcome in clinical trials and the comparison between and within centers over time [21].

The NICHD together with the National Heart, Lung, and Blood Institute held a workshop in 2000 entitled, "From BPD to CLD: Emergence of a New Disease," in which a severity-based definition of BPD was proposed [22]. Criteria for mild, moderate, and severe BPD were defined for infants with gestational age less than 32 weeks, who had received oxygen therapy, for at least 28 days and were assessed at either the time of discharge or at 36 weeks postmenstrual age, whichever came first. A diagnosis of mild BPD was assigned to infants who at time of assessment were in room air, moderate BPD to those who were in less than 30% oxygen, and severe BPD to those needing at least 30% oxygen and/or positive pressure ventilation or continuous positive airway pressure. The predictive validity of these proposed severity-based definitions for BPD on pulmonary, neurodevelopmental, and growth outcomes at 18 to 22 months' corrected age was reported in 2005 [23]. As the severity of BPD increased, the incidence of neurodevelopmental or sensory impairment significantly increased. Pulmonary outcomes related to use of medication and rehospitalization for pulmonary causes as well as growth outcomes were also significantly adversely affected as the severity of BPD increased. The authors concluded that these severity-based diagnostic criteria for BPD identify a spectrum of risk for adverse pulmonary and neurodevelopmental outcomes in early infancy more accurately than other definitions. A similar conclusion was drawn in a report from a single site whereby the new system for grading the severity of BPD offered a better description of underlying pulmonary disease and correlated well with the infant's maturity, growth, and overall severity of illness [24].

In 2006, the NICHD published the summary proceedings from the Bronchopulmonary Dysplasia Group [25]. Similar to the 2000 NICHD/National Heart, Lung, and Blood Institute workshop, the goal of this working group was to develop definitions of BPD that would reflect disease severity. The NICHD definition was stratified by postmenstrual age, with different end points for infants born before 32 weeks and those born at or beyond 32 weeks. For infants less than 32 weeks gestation, mild BPD was defined as an oxygen requirement for the first 28 days but in room air at 36 weeks postmenstrual age. Moderate BPD was defined as an oxygen requirement for the first 28 days and a need for a FiO_2 less than 0.3 at 36 weeks, whereas severe BPD was defined as an oxygen requirement for the first 28 days and FiO_2 need of at least 0.3 and continuous positive airway pressure or mechanical ventilation at 36 weeks postmenstrual age. For more mature infants born at or beyond 32 weeks, the definition of BPD was adjusted for the end point of 56 days rather than 36 weeks. The need to assess the severity of BPD using standardized definitions becomes apparent when the association between severe BPD and poor long-term neurodevelopmental outcomes is taken into account. For example, a relationship between prolonged ventilation of over 60 days and death or neurodevelopmental impairment at 18 months was recently reported among 5364 infants who weighed between 501 and 1000 g in the NICHD Network database between 1995 and 1998 [26]. When standardized definitions of disease severity are combined with the physiologic definition of BPD in selected infants with oxygen saturation monitoring (Fig. 1), they should provide objective and validated information on the severity of this clinical outcome and a reliable means to compare data across centers and assess the impact of interventions [25].

Although these studies have brought objectivity to the definition of BPD, during this transition phase, there has been considerable confusion and ambiguity for both investigators and clinicians. How many definitions of BPD are needed or helpful? Which definition is optimal for a randomized clinical trial, or for patient care? Is it appropriate to adopt a one-size-fits-all approach to oxygen saturation targets? Although individual adjustments in targeted oxygen saturations will need to be made based on the underlying cardiopulmonary pathology, for the purposes of clinical trials design and benchmarking, the authors believe the use of an objective, well-defined definition, such as the physiologic definition, combined with criteria to grade BPD severity as suggested by the NIH Consensus definitions will prove optimal (see Fig. 1). Together, they fulfill most needs for both clinicians and investigators.

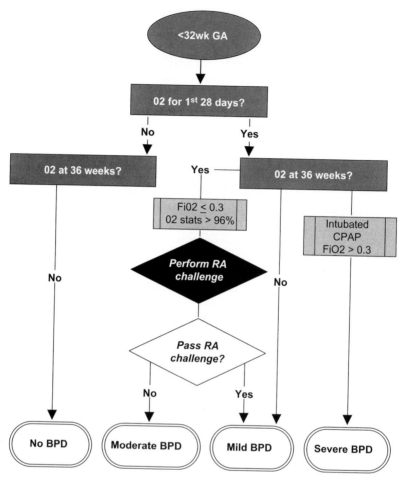

Fig. 1. Proposed criteria for defining and categorizing the severity of BPD. BPD is diagnosed in any infant less than 32 weeks gestation with a history of needing supplemental oxygen during the first 28 days. Disease severity is determined at 36 weeks postmenstrual age. Severe BPD is a designation reserved for infants who at 36 weeks are receiving mechanical ventilation, continuous positive airway pressure, or require supplemental oxygen FiO_2 greater than 0.3. A room air challenge test with a stepwise reduction in oxygen concentration to 0.21 is given to any infant whose FiO_2 is less than or equal to 0.3 with adequate saturations at 36 weeks postmenstrual age. Infants who do not maintain adequate saturations at a FiO_2 of 0.21 are considered to have moderate BPD. Mild BPD is diagnosed at 36 weeks in those who pass the room air challenge test or who, subsequent to day 28 of life, weaned to and remain in room air at 36 weeks. Note: For infants born beyond 32 weeks gestation, the same criteria are used but the determination of disease severity is made at 56 days rather than 36 weeks. CPAP, continuous positive airway pressure; GA, gestational age; RA, room air.

Randomized controlled trials: the great melting pot of neonatology?

Even a standardized and universally accepted definition is not likely to eliminate the variability among centers or individual patients, or overcome the sample size problem faced by the neonatology clinical trials community. Although large neonatal networks provide more power to determine the efficacy of an intervention, center-to-center variation in populations and care practices, and therefore in outcomes, can overwhelm the effect of an intervention [27]. Large differences in outcomes such as BPD, retinopathy of prematurity, or necrotizing enterocolitis among centers suggest differences in care practices and/or in neonatal populations that will remain even after standardized definitions are accepted and adopted. The upshot is that large treatment effects are required to demonstrate either benefit or harm of an intervention. This has perhaps been best demonstrated by the trials conducted by the NICHD Neonatal Network, whereby reported BPD rates varied between 5% and 76% and neurodevelopmental impairment (cerebral palsy or developmental index score less than 70) varied between 25% and 69% [28]. Thus, the power and advantage of large numbers may be offset by center-to-center variability in outcomes, so that the effect of an intervention would be difficult to detect [27].

On the other hand, randomization by center balances these differences and compensates for the variation. Also, it can be argued that the variation within a network reflects the variation that will inevitably be seen in the real world, and thus is a strength rather than a weakness. This is the difference between effectiveness (as shown in a pristine RCT with strict eligibility criteria) and efficacy (the impact observed when a new or changed practice is applied in the real world). Efficacy rarely attains the level of effectiveness demonstrated in clinical trials.

Small trials searching for a cure for BPD are bound to yield disappointing results. Given the complexity of this disease, it is unlikely that any one therapy will have a large treatment effect, and detection of small—but significant—reductions in disease incidence and severity will require large trials [29]. One of the few therapies reported to exert a positive impact on BPD is vitamin A [30]. Given over the first 4 weeks of life, vitamin A supplements significantly increased survival without BPD compared to placebo. The absolute reduction in death or BPD was 7%, with one case of BPD prevented for every 14 to 15 infants treated with vitamin A. Unfortunately, the neonatology community has been slow to embrace therapies with small treatment effects [29].

The great diversity of neonatal clinical care is rarely appreciated outside of our own community. This applies not only to our individualized local care practices, but also to our patient population. This fact is particularly relevant to intervention trials for BPD. BPD is a complex disease of altered lung developmental processes. Not only must our clinical trials strategy take into account differences in the severity of the outcome, but we must consider that molecular and cellular mechanisms leading to BPD may be different at different gestational ages and the stage of saccular lung development at which the prenatal and postnatal insults occur. It is likely that these molecular processes are modified by the types of exogenous stimuli (inflammation, hyperoxia, mechanical shear stress related to tidal ventilation) that clinicians have long recognized as being associated with BPD. Thus, the response to an intervention may differ depending on the predominant mechanism driving altered lung developmental processes in that patient, and the timing and duration of the insult and the intervention. We, as pediatricians, fundamentally understand that neonates are not just small adults. It is time to profess that a 23 to 25-week–gestation preterm infant may be fundamentally different than a 26- to 28-week–gestation infant and design our enrollment stratification and data analysis accordingly. Otherwise, we may not only fail to recognize a therapy that is beneficial for a subset of our patients, but we may erroneously endorse an intervention that is harmful to another.

Focusing in on the future

We are currently blessed and cursed with a plethora of definitions for BPD, leaving us temporarily in limbo. However, we have faced this dilemma before. As a subspecialty, we have adapted to meet the needs of our changing patient population and our research community by shifting from the Northway et al [31] definition (based on radiologic, clinical, and pathologic criteria) to the 1979 Bancalari et al [32] definition (an oxygen requirement at 28 days), and then, with relative ease to the 1988 Shennan et al [33] definition (an oxygen requirement at 36 weeks). Once the integration of the physiologic definition of BPD with the NIH consensus definitions of disease severity has been validated, the authors predict there will be rapid and fairly uniform adoption of a standardized set of definitions. The physiologic definition will primarily inform the consensus definition by splitting patients between the mild and moderate BPD categories (see Fig. 1). Patients who required oxygen for the first 28 days, remain on or develop an oxygen requirement at 36 weeks, and meet the criteria for room air challenge, will be said to have mild BPD if they pass the challenge, and moderate BPD if they fail the challenge. In this way, an objective measure of disease will be combined with a measure of the severity of the illness.

In the future, it would be desirable to directly assess an infant's functional respiratory status with bedside pulmonary function tests. Such tests are currently feasible in intubated neonates and in older nonintubated infants as young as 4 months of age and have revolutionized the care of neonates with cystic fibrosis [34]. Unfortunately, the currently available tests for nonintubated older infants require sedation and are appropriate only for those over 4 months of age. It would be highly desirable to develop such techniques to study nonintubated convalescent premature infants in the future.

Enhanced capabilities to assess infant pulmonary function will hopefully also be accompanied by the development of noninvasive, sophisticated imaging techniques to study pulmonary structure. This is another innovation that has improved the care of infants who have cystic fibrosis [35]. The use of advanced imaging systems such as high-resolution computerized tomography and dynamic imaging magnetic resonance has allowed detailed imaging of the airways and has improved the understanding of the pathophysiologic derangements in lung disease. Such understanding would improve our ability to tailor treatments to the infant who has bronchopulmonary dysplasia and to integrate knowledge of structure with knowledge of function.

Our current concepts of long-term outcomes may be a bit short-sighted. In the authors' myopic view of the NICU, where a 3-month hospital stay is not unusual, anything beyond discharge seems to meet the definition of long-term. We need to partner with pediatric and adult pulmonologists and school psychologists to begin to address the relevant and truly long-term effects of BPD. What will be the impact of smoking on the health and longevity of survivors of prematurity and BPD? How will aging impact the aberrant pulmonary vascular and alveolar architecture of the BPD lung? What degree of pulmonary developmental arrest can be overcome, and what are the life-long susceptibilities of these individuals? Long-term cohort evaluations are needed to assess these later outcomes.

Summary

Future gains in neonatal intensive care are unlikely to be as spectacular as those achieved in the past two decades, especially with regard to mortality [36]. Although the neonatal community can take pride in past accomplishments that have contributed to improved survival for preterm infants, neonatology is infamous for the adoption of new therapies into wide-spread practice before efficacy and safety have been rigorously evaluated and validated [29]. This legacy demands that we adopt a more scientific approach to the implementation of new therapies and practices. A long history of therapeutic misadventures has convinced our subspecialty of the need to shift the focus of clinical trials from short-term efficacy to long-term safety. A much higher bar has been set than ever before for the introduction of new therapies into the NICU. Adoption of new practices and interventions must be based on strong evidence from clinical trials that have been powered to address the possibility of harm as well as the prospect of benefit. The goals of the neonatology clinical research community in the coming decade must be the evaluation of new and established interventions that will reduce morbidity and enhance long-term quality of life.

References

[1] Suresh GK, Soll RF. Overview of surfactant replacement trials. J Perinatol 2005;25(Suppl 2): S40–4.

[2] Soll RF. Multiple versus single dose natural surfactant extract for severe neonatal respiratory distress syndrome. Cochrane Database Syst Rev 2000;2:CD000141.

[3] Soll RF, Morley CJ. Prophylactic versus selective use of surfactant for preventing morbidity and mortality in preterm infants. Cochrane Database Syst Rev 2000;2:CD000510.

[4] Yost CC, Soll RF. Early versus delayed selective surfactant treatment for neonatal respiratory distress syndrome. Cochrane Database Syst Rev 2000;2:CD001456.

[5] Soll RF, Blanco F. Natural surfactant extract versus synthetic surfactant for neonatal respiratory distress syndrome. Cochrane Database Syst Rev 2000;2:CD000144.

[6] Morley C, Davis P. Surfactant treatment for premature lung disorders: a review of best practices in 2002. Paediatr Respir Rev 2004;5(Suppl A):S299–304.

[7] Sinn JK, Ward MC, Henderson-Smart DJ. Developmental outcome of preterm infants after surfactant therapy: systematic review of randomized controlled trials. J Paediatr Child Health 2002;38(6):597–600.

[8] Moya FR, Gadzinowski J, Bancalari E, et al. A multicenter, randomized, masked, comparison trial of lucinactant, colfosceril palmitate, and beractant for the prevention of respiratory distress syndrome among very preterm infants. Pediatrics 2005;115(4):1018–29.

[9] Sinha SK, Lacaze-Masmonteil T, Valls i Soler A, et al. A multicenter, randomized, controlled trial of lucinactant versus poractant alfa among very premature infants at high risk for respiratory distress syndrome. Pediatrics 2005;115(4):1030–8.

[10] Horbar JD, Soll RF, Sutherland JM, et al. A multicenter randomized, placebo-controlled trial of surfactant therapy for respiratory distress syndrome. N Engl J Med 1989;320(15): 959–65.

[11] Collaborative European Multicenter Study Group. Surfactant replacement therapy for severe neonatal respiratory distress syndrome: an international randomized clinical trial. Pediatrics 1988;82(5):683–91.

[12] Horbar JD, Carpenter JH, Buzas J, et al. Timing of initial surfactant treatment for infants 23 to 29 weeks' gestation: is routine practice evidence based? Pediatrics 2004;113(6): 1593–602.

[13] Finer NN, Carlo WA, Duara S, et al. Delivery room continuous positive airway pressure/ positive end-expiratory pressure in extremely low birth weight infants: a feasibility trial. Pediatrics 2004;114(3):651–7.

[14] Sandri F, Ancora G, Lanzoni A, et al. Prophylactic nasal continuous positive airways pressure in newborns of 28-31 weeks gestation: multicentre randomised controlled clinical trial. Arch Dis Child Fetal Neonatal Ed 2004;89(5):F394–8.

[15] Kinsella JP, Greenough A, Abman SH. Bronchopulmonary dysplasia. Lancet 2006;367: 1421–31.

[16] Doyle LW, Faber B, Callanan C, et al. Bronchopulmonary dysplasia in very low birth weight subjects and lung function in late adolescence. Pediatrics 2006;118(1):108–13.

[17] Doyle LW, the Victorian Infant Collaborative Study Group. Respiratory function at age 8-9 years in extremely low birthweight/very preterm children born in Victoria in 1991-1992. Pediatr Pulmonol 2006;41(6):570–6.

[18] Dammann O, Leviton A, Bartels DB, et al. Lung and brain damage in preterm newborns. Are they related? How? Why? Biol Neonate 2004;85(4):305–13.

[19] O'Shea TM. Cerebral palsy in very preterm infants: new epidemiological insights. Ment Retard Dev Disabil Res Rev 2002;8:135–45.

[20] Walsh MC, Wilson-Costello D, Zadell A, et al. Safety, reliability, and validity of a physiologic definition of bronchopulmonary dysplasia. J Perinatol 2003;23(6):451–6.

[21] Walsh MC, Yao Q, Gettner P, et al. Impact of a physiologic definition on bronchopulmonary dysplasia rates. Pediatrics 2004;114(5):1305–11.

[22] Jobe AH, Bancalari E. Bronchopulmonary dysplasia. Am J Respir Crit Care Med 2001;163: 1723–9.

[23] Ehrenkrantz R, Walsh MC, Vohr B, et al. Validation of the National Institutes of Health consensus definition of bronchopulmonary dysplasia. Pediatrics 2005;116:1353–60.

[24] Sahni R, Ammari A, Suri MS, et al. Is the new definition of bronchopulmonary dysplasia more useful? J Perinatol 2005;25(1):41–6.

[25] Walsh MC, Szefler S, Davis J, et al. Summary proceedings from the Bronchopulmonary Dysplasia Group. Pediatrics 2006;117(3):S52–6.

[26] Walsh MC, Morris BH, Wrage L, et al. Extremely low birthweight neonates with protracted ventilation: mortality and 18-month neurodevelopmental outcomes. J Pediatr 2005;146(6): 798–804.

[27] Welty SE. Critical issues with clinical research in children: the example of premature infants. Toxicol Appl Pharmacol 2005;207(2 Suppl):673–8.

[28] Vohr BR, Wright LL, Dusick AM, et al. Center differences and outcomes of extremely low birth weight infants. Pediatrics 2004;113(4):781–9.

[29] Aschner JL. Non-pulmonary therapy in the NICU. Pediatr Pulmonol 2004;26:162–5.

[30] Tyson JE, Wright LL, Oh W, et al. Vitamin A supplementation for extremely-low-birthweight infants. N Engl J Med 1999;340(25):1962–8.

[31] Northway WH Jr, Rosan RC, Porter DY. Pulmonary disease following respirator therapy of hyaline-membrane disease. Bronchopulmonary dysplasia. N Engl J Med 1967;276(7): 357–68.

[32] Bancalari E, Abdenour GE, Feller R, et al. Bronchopulmonary dysplasia: clinical presentation. J Pediatr 1979;95(5 Pt 2):819–23.

[33] Shennan AT, Dunn MS, Ohlsson A, et al. Abnormal pulmonary outcomes in premature infants: prediction from oxygen requirement in the neonatal period. Pediatrics 1988;82(4): 527–32.

[34] Davis S, Jones M, Kisling J, et al. Comparison of normal infants and infants with cystic fibrosis using forced expiratory flows breathing air and heliox. Pediatr Pulmonol 2001;31(1): 17–23.

[35] Martinez TM, Llapur CJ, Williams TH, et al. High-resolution computed tomography imaging of airway disease in infants with cystic fibrosis. Am J Respir Crit Care Med 2005;172: 1133–8.

[36] Harrold J, Schmidt B. Evidence-based neonatology: making a difference beyond discharge from the neonatal nursery. Curr Opin Pediatr 2002;14(2):165–9.

ELSEVIER
SAUNDERS

Clin Perinatol 34 (2007) 219–226

CLINICS IN
PERINATOLOGY

Index

Note: Page numbers of article titles are in **boldface** type.

0095-5108/07/$ - see front matter © 2007 Elsevier Inc. All rights reserved.
doi:10.1016/S0095-5108(07)00018-8

perinatology.theclinics.com

Moving?

Make sure your subscription moves with you!

To notify us of your new address, find your **Clinics Account Number** (located on your mailing label above your name), and contact customer service at:

E-mail: elspcs@elsevier.com

800-654-2452 (subscribers in the U.S. & Canada)
407-345-4000 (subscribers outside of the U.S. & Canada)

Fax number: 407-363-9661

Elsevier Periodicals Customer Service
6277 Sea Harbor Drive
Orlando, FL 32887-4800

*To ensure uninterrupted delivery of your subscription, please notify us at least 4 weeks in advance of move.